The 90 Day Transformation: A Journey To Weight Loss Without The Gym

DISCLAIMER

The information contained in this resource is general in nature and for informative purposes only.

The Author assumes no responsibility whatsoever, under any circumstances, for any actions taken as a result of the information contained herein.

You are required to seek professional help if needed.

Before this document is duplicated or reproduced in any manner, the publisher's consent must be gained. Therefore, the contents within can neither be stored electronically, transferred, nor kept in a database.

Neither in Part nor full can the document be copied, scanned, faxed, or retained without approval from the publisher or creator.

Preface

In a world where the quest for health and fitness often leads us through the revolving doors of gyms, we forget that the key to wellness lies not just in the clanking of weights but in the simplicity of our daily choices. "The 90-Day Transformation: A Journey to Weight loss Without the Gym" is a testament to the power of transformation that resides within each of us.7

This book is not just a guide; it's a journey. A journey that begins not with heavy lifting, but with lifting the veil on the myths that surround weight loss. It's a path that doesn't require a gym membership but does demand a commitment to change – change in the way we eat, think, and live.

Over the next 90 days, you'll discover that losing weight is more about gaining insight into your body and mind than about shedding pounds. You'll learn that your kitchen can be as effective as any gym and that your willpower is the strongest muscle you can flex.

As you turn these pages, you'll find strategies, tips, and a day-by-day plan that will guide you through a transformation that is not only physical but also mental and emotional. You'll emerge not just lighter in body, but also enriched in spirit and knowledge.

Welcome to the revolution. A revolution that doesn't ask for a gym, but for your determination to take the first step and keep moving forward.

Leo Chambers

Contents

2. **Fueling Your Transformation: Effective Nutrition Strategies For Weight Loss Without The Gym**
    - *Balanced Eating*: The Art of Portion Control And Nutrient Harmony For Weight Lose Without the Gym.
    - *Healthy Snacking*: Conquering Cravings With nutritious and Delicious snack options Without the Gym.
    - *Intermittent Fasting*: Exploring Alternative eating pattern for weight loss without the Gym.
3. **Unleash Your Inner Athlete: Effective Home Workouts For Weight Loss Without The Gym**
    - *Bodyweight Exercises*: Master effective bodyweight exercises for strength and toning.
    - *HIIT (High-Intensity Interval Training)*: Create a home HIIT routine.
    - *Yoga and Pilates*: Learn about low-impact workouts for flexibility and muscle endurance.
4. **Mindset and Motivation: Fueling Your 90-Day Weight Loss Journey**

- *Mindful Eating:* Cultivate awareness around food choices For Lasting Weight Loss
    - *Positive Affirmations:* Boost motivation and self-belief For Weight Loss Success Without The Gym
    - *Overcoming Plateaus:* Strategies to break through weight loss Stalls.

5. **Sleep and Recovery: The Unsung Heroes Of Weight Loss**
    - *Quality Sleep:* The Powerhouse Behind weight loss.
    - *Rest Days:* The importance of allowing your body to rebuild and recharge.
    - *Stress Management:* Techniques to reduce stress-related weight gain.

6. **Tracking Progress and Adjustments: Mastering Your 90 Day Weight Loss Journey**
    - *Food Journaling:* Keep track of your meals and progress.
    - *Weekly Assessments:* Evaluating your weight loss journey and making Adjustments.
    - *Adaptability:* The Key to sustainable weight loss.

7. Weight Loss Supplements: A Critical Examination

Acknowledgement

About the Author

Introduction

In a world where the hustle and bustle of daily life often leave us with little time for ourselves, the quest for health and fitness can seem like a distant dream. But what if I told you that the secret to shedding those extra pounds and transforming your body didn't require a gym membership or expensive equipment? What if all it took was a commitment to yourself and a journey of self-discovery?

"The 90-Day Transformation: A Journey to Weight Loss Without the Gym" is not just a book; it's a companion on your path to a healthier you. Over the next three months, you'll embark on an adventure that will challenge your perceptions of weight loss and fitness. You'll learn that the power to change lies within you, in the choices you make every day, and in the small steps you take towards a larger goal.

This book is your guide through a forest of misconceptions and a sea of false promises. It's a beacon of hope and a testament to the fact that you can achieve your weight loss goals. So, let's turn the page and begin the first chapter of your transformation story, where every day is a new opportunity to become the best version of yourself—no gym required.

Over the next 90 days, you'll learn how to harness the power of nutrition, effective at-home workouts, and the psychology of weight loss to create lasting change. Whether you're a busy professional, a stay-at-home parent, or someone who simply prefers the privacy of their own space, this book is tailored for you.

Embark on this journey with an open mind and a committed heart, and watch as you transform not only your body but also your relationship with health and fitness. Let's redefine what's possible and make the next 90 days the most impactful of your life.

Chapter 1
Understanding the Basics

Introduction to Weight Loss

Weight loss is a journey that involves a comprehensive understanding of your body, nutrition, and lifestyle habits. It's not just about shedding pounds but about making sustainable changes that lead to a healthier you. This chapter will explore the fundamental principles of weight loss, debunk common myths, and set the stage for a transformative 90-day journey.

The Science of Weight Loss

To lose weight, you must create a calorie deficit, which means burning more calories than you consume. This can be achieved through dietary changes, increased physical activity, or a combination of both. We'll delve into the science behind calorie counting, the role of macronutrients, and how your body metabolizes food to use it as energy.

Setting Realistic Goals

Setting achievable goals is crucial for weight loss success. We'll discuss how to set SMART (Specific, Measurable, Achievable, Relevant, Time-bound) goals that motivate you without setting you up for disappointment. You'll learn how to track your progress and adjust your goals as you move forward.

Understanding Your Body Type

Everyone's body is unique, and understanding your body type—ectomorph, mesomorph, or endomorph—can help tailor your weight loss plan. This section will explain the characteristics of each body type and provide tips for effective weight loss strategies that align with your natural physique.

Nutrition Fundamentals

Proper nutrition is the cornerstone of weight loss. We'll cover the basics of a balanced diet, the importance of micronutrients, and how to read food labels. You'll also learn about portion control and how to make smart food choices that support your weight loss goals.

The Role of Hydration

Hydration plays a vital role in weight loss and overall health. This section will highlight the benefits of staying hydrated, how much water you should drink daily, and the impact of hydration on metabolism and satiety.

Sleep and Weight Loss

Adequate sleep is often overlooked in weight loss plans. We'll explore the connection between sleep and weight management, including how sleep deprivation can affect your appetite, hormones, and energy levels.

Stress Management

Stress can sabotage your weight loss efforts by triggering emotional eating and slowing down your metabolism. This section will provide strategies for managing stress, including mindfulness, relaxation techniques, and the importance of self-care.

Building a Support System

Having a support system can greatly enhance your weight loss journey. We'll discuss how to build a network of friends, family, or online communities that encourage and motivate you. You'll learn how to seek support when you need it and how to deal with unsupportive environments.

Preparing for the Journey

Before embarking on your 90-day weight loss journey, it's important to prepare mentally and physically. This section will guide you through setting up your environment for success, including meal planning, scheduling time for physical activity, and creating a positive mindset.

This content serves as a comprehensive guide to the basics of weight loss, providing you with the knowledge and tools needed to begin your journey.

Remember, weight loss is a personal experience, and what works for one person may not work for another. It's important to listen to your body and make adjustments to your plan as needed. Good luck on your 90-day journey to a healthier you!

Calorie Deficit: The Math Behind the Burn

Dreaming of a slimmer you but gym memberships and intense workouts don't quite fit your style? You're in luck! Creating a calorie deficit, the core principle behind weight loss, can be achieved without ever stepping foot in a gym. This chapter dives deep into understanding calorie deficit and equips you with effective strategies to achieve it, paving the way for a healthy and sustainable weight loss journey in just 90 days.

Understanding Calorie Deficit: The Math Behind the Burn

Imagine your body as a burning furnace. Food fuels this furnace, providing energy for daily activities. Calorie deficit simply means burning more calories than you consume. When this happens, your body dips into stored energy (fat) to compensate for the shortfall, leading to weight loss.

Calculating Your Calorie Needs

The first step is figuring out your body's daily calorie needs. This magic number represents the amount of energy your body burns to maintain its current weight. There are two key components:
- **Basal Metabolic Rate (BMR):** The minimum calories your body needs for basic functions like breathing and circulation.
- **Activity Level:** The calories burned through daily activities.

Several online calculators or apps can estimate your BMR based on factors like age, weight, height, and gender. Once you have your BMR, consider your activity level and use the following multipliers:
- Sedentary (little to no exercise): BMR x 1.2
- Lightly active (1-3 days of exercise): BMR x 1.375
- Moderately active (3-5 days): BMR x 1.55
- Very active (6-7 days): BMR x 1.725
- Extremely active (athletes): BMR x 1.9

Creating a Sustainable Calorie Deficit

Aiming for a drastic calorie deficit might seem tempting, but it's often unsustainable and counterproductive. Here's a safe and effective approach:

1. **Start Small:** Begin by creating a deficit of 300-500 calories from your calculated daily needs. This translates to a weight loss of 0.5-1 pound per week, a healthy and realistic goal.
2. **Track Your Calories:** Food journaling or using calorie-tracking apps helps you stay mindful of your intake. It highlights areas for adjustments and keeps you accountable.

Diet Strategies for a Calorie Deficit

Now comes the fun part: revamping your diet for success! Here are some key strategies:

- **Portion Control:** Use smaller plates and bowls to subconsciously reduce portion sizes.
- **Focus on Whole Foods:** Prioritize fruits, vegetables, whole grains, and lean proteins. These are nutrient-dense and keep you feeling fuller for longer.

- **Fiber Power**: Load up on fiber-rich foods like fruits, vegetables, and whole grains. They promote satiety and aid digestion.
- **Protein Prowess**: Include protein sources like chicken, fish, beans, and lentils in your meals. Protein boosts metabolism and helps preserve muscle mass during weight loss.
- **Hydration Hero**: Drink plenty of water throughout the day. It curbs cravings, aids digestion, and keeps you feeling full.
- **Beware of Hidden Calories**: Limit sugary drinks, processed foods, and unhealthy fats. These are calorie-dense and often lack essential nutrients.
- **Mindful Eating**: Savor your food, chew thoroughly, and avoid distractions while eating. This promotes mindful consumption and helps you recognize satiety cues.

Non-Gym Activities to Boost Your Deficit

While the gym isn't mandatory, incorporating some physical activity into your routine can accelerate your weight loss journey. Here are some excellent options:

- **NEAT Hacks**: Increase your Non-Exercise Activity Thermogenesis (NEAT) by fidgeting, taking the stairs, parking further away, or doing household chores with more vigor.

- **Brisk Walking:** This simple activity burns calories and is a great way to incorporate movement into your daily routine.
- **Home Workouts:** Numerous free online workout videos cater to all fitness levels. Find something you enjoy and can do at home.
- **Active Hobbies:** Explore activities like dancing, swimming, cycling, or hiking. They keep things fun while burning calories.

Remember: Consistency is key! Aim for small, sustainable changes that you can maintain over the long term. Celebrate your progress, don't get discouraged by setbacks, and enjoy the journey to a healthier, slimmer you!

Unleashing Your Inner Furnace: Natural Ways to Boost Metabolism for Weight Loss (Without the Gym)

In your 90-day journey to weight loss without the gym, understanding and optimizing your metabolism is crucial. This chapter delves into the fascinating world of metabolism, exploring natural strategies to turn your body into a more efficient calorie-burning machine, paving the way for successful weight loss.

What is Metabolism and Why Does it Matter?
Imagine your body as a complex engine. Metabolism refers to the set of processes by which your body converts food into energy. This energy fuels everything you do, from breathing and thinking to walking and exercising. The higher your metabolic rate, the more calories you burn at rest and during activity.
Here's why understanding metabolism is essential for weight loss:

- **Burning More Calories:** A higher metabolic rate means your body burns more calories throughout the day, even when you're not actively exercising. This creates a calorie deficit, the core principle behind weight loss.
- **Preserving Muscle Mass:** Muscle tissue burns more calories than fat tissue, even at rest. By boosting your metabolism, you can help preserve muscle mass, which is crucial for long-term weight management and overall health.
- **Enhanced Energy Levels:** An efficient metabolism ensures your body has the energy it needs to function optimally. You'll

feel more energized throughout the day,
making it easier to stay active and support
your weight loss goals.

Natural Ways to Ignite Your Metabolism

The good news is that several natural strategies
can help you elevate your metabolism and
accelerate your weight loss journey, all without
requiring a gym membership. Let's explore these
strategies in detail:

1. **Protein Powerhouse:**
   - **The Science:** Protein has a thermic effect,
     meaning your body burns more calories
     digesting and absorbing it compared to carbs
     or fats. This translates to a slight metabolic
     boost.
   - **The Strategy:** Aim to include a source of
     lean protein in every meal and snack. Opt for
     options like chicken, fish, beans, lentils, low-
     fat dairy, and tofu.
   - **Bonus Tip:** Spread your protein intake
     throughout the day to maintain muscle mass
     and keep your metabolism humming.
2. **Fiber Fiesta:**
   - **The Science:** Fiber keeps you feeling fuller
     for longer, reducing calorie intake and

potentially boosting metabolism through increased thermogenesis (heat production) during digestion.

- **The Strategy:** Load up on high-fiber foods like fruits, vegetables, whole grains, and legumes. Aim for at least 25-35 grams of fiber daily.
- **Bonus Tip:** Start your day with a fiber-rich breakfast, like oatmeal with berries, to keep you feeling satisfied and curb cravings throughout the morning.

3. **Spice Up Your Life:**
   - **The Science:** Chili peppers contain capsaicin, a compound that may increase thermogenesis and slightly boost metabolism for a short period.
   - **The Strategy:** Add chili peppers, cayenne pepper, or even black pepper to your meals. Experiment with different spices to find flavors you enjoy.
   - **Bonus Tip:** While the effect of capsaicin is modest, it can add a flavorful kick to your meals and potentially enhance satiety.

4. **Green Tea Goodness:**
   - **The Science:** Green tea contains caffeine and epigallocatechin gallate (EGCG), a

compound that may promote thermogenesis and fat burning.

- **The Strategy**: Enjoy 2-3 cups of green tea daily. Choose loose leaf or bag varieties, depending on your preference.
- **Bonus Tip**: Experiment with different green tea flavors like jasmine or lemon to find one you enjoy. Remember, consistency is key!

5. **Sleep for Success**:
  - **The Science**: When sleep-deprived, your body produces more ghrelin (the hunger hormone) and less leptin (the satiety hormone), leading to increased cravings and potential weight gain. Adequate sleep may also regulate hormones that influence metabolism.
  - **The Strategy**: Aim for 7-8 hours of quality sleep each night. Establish a regular sleep schedule and create a relaxing bedtime routine.
  - **Bonus Tip**: Create a sleep-conducive environment by keeping your bedroom dark, quiet, and cool.

6. **Hydration Hero**:
  - **The Science**: Dehydration can slow down your metabolism. Water plays a crucial role

in various bodily functions, including digestion and nutrient absorption.

- **The Strategy:** Drink plenty of water throughout the day. Aim for eight glasses of water daily, adjusting based on your activity level and climate.
- **Bonus Tip:** Infuse your water with slices of fruit, cucumber, or herbs for a refreshing and flavorful twist.

7. **Mindful Eating Magic:**

- **The Science:** Mindful eating practices encourage you to slow down, savor your food, and pay attention to the body's hunger and satiety cues. This can help prevent overeating and support a healthy metabolism.
- **The Strategy:** Practice mindful eating techniques like:
    - **Eating slowly and chewing thoroughly.**
    - **Turning off distractions while eating.**
    - **Focusing on the taste and texture of your food.**
    - **Stopping when you're comfortably full, not stuffed.**
- **Bonus Tip:** Mindful eating takes practice, but it can become a powerful tool for weight management and overall well-being.

8. **Strength Training Surprise:**

- **The Science**: While not requiring a gym membership, strength training, even bodyweight exercises at home, can build muscle mass. Muscle burns more calories at rest than fat, leading to a slight but sustained increase in metabolism.
- **The Strategy**: Aim for 2-3 strength training sessions per week, targeting all major muscle groups. Utilize bodyweight exercises like squats, lunges, push-ups, planks, and rows.
- **Bonus Tip**: You can gradually increase the difficulty of these exercises over time to keep challenging your muscles and maximizing metabolic benefits.

9. HIIT it Hard (Even at Home):

- **The Science**: High-Intensity Interval Training (HIIT) alternates between short bursts of intense activity and periods of rest. This style of training can elevate your metabolism for a longer period after the workout, even compared to moderate-intensity exercise.
- **The Strategy**: Find HIIT workouts you can do at home. Many free online resources offer bodyweight HIIT routines requiring minimal to no equipment.

- **Bonus Tip:** Start with shorter HIIT sessions (10-15 minutes) and gradually increase the duration and intensity as your fitness level improves.

10. Manage Stress, Maximize Results:

- **The Science:** Chronic stress elevates cortisol levels, a hormone that can promote fat storage and hinder weight loss. Reducing stress may indirectly support a healthy metabolism.
- **The Strategy:** Find healthy stress-management techniques that work for you. Consider relaxation techniques like deep breathing, meditation, yoga, or spending time in nature.
- **Bonus Tip:** Prioritize activities you enjoy and find calming. Regularly incorporating stress-management practices can make a significant difference in your overall well-being.

Remember: Consistency is Key!

While each of these strategies can contribute to boosting your metabolism, the key to success lies in consistency. Aim to incorporate these practices into your daily routine for optimal results. Don't expect overnight miracles; focus on gradual, sustainable changes that you can maintain over the long term.

Additional Considerations:
- **Individual Variability**: Metabolism can vary significantly between individuals due to factors like genetics, age, and body composition.
- **Underlying Conditions**: Certain medical conditions can affect metabolism. Consult with your doctor if you have any concerns.
- **Calorie Balance**: Remember, creating a calorie deficit through a combination of healthy eating and physical activity remains the cornerstone of weight loss.

By implementing these natural strategies, you can unlock your body's full metabolic potential and accelerate your weight loss journey in the comfort of your own home. Embrace a holistic approach to well-being, focusing on not just weight loss but also on cultivating healthy habits that will empower you to achieve and maintain lasting results.

Setting Realistic Goals: Establishing Achievable Weight Loss Targets for Your 90-Day Transformation (Without the Gym)

Embarking on a weight loss journey is an exciting step towards a healthier you. However, setting unrealistic goals can lead to frustration and discouragement. This subchapter equips you with the tools and strategies to establish achievable weight loss targets for your 90-day transformation, setting the stage for sustainable success without requiring a gym membership.

Understanding Realistic Weight Loss
While the title of your book mentions achieving results in 90 days, it's crucial to understand healthy and realistic weight loss expectations. Aiming for drastic weight loss within a short timeframe is often unsustainable and potentially unhealthy. Let's explore some key principles:

- **Safe and Effective:** Losing 1-2 pounds per week is considered safe and effective for long-term weight management. This translates to a total weight loss of 4-8 pounds in 90 days, a realistic and achievable target.
- **Focus on Habits:** Instead of solely focusing on the number on the scale, prioritize

building healthy habits that will support lasting weight loss. This includes mindful eating, portion control, regular physical activity, and adequate sleep.

Calculating Your Healthy Weight Loss Range
Here's a step-by-step approach to determine your personalized healthy weight loss range for the 90-day program:
1. **Body Mass Index (BMI):** This is a simple calculation that provides a general idea of your weight status. You can find numerous online BMI calculators or calculate it manually using your weight and height.
2. **Healthy Weight Range:** Based on your BMI, identify your healthy weight range. Reputable health organizations like the National Institutes of Health (NIH) provide BMI charts with corresponding weight ranges.
3. **Current Weight:** Knowing your current weight is crucial. Weigh yourself accurately and consistently, ideally first thing in the morning after using the restroom.
4. **Realistic Target:** Considering your BMI, healthy weight range, and overall health goals, set a realistic target weight for the

end of your 90-day program. Aim to lose 1-2 pounds per week, falling within the 4-8 pound total weight loss range.

Remember: Consulting with a healthcare professional or registered dietitian can provide personalized guidance on safe and effective weight loss goals, especially if you have any underlying health conditions.

Setting SMART Goals for Weight Loss
SMART goals are a powerful tool for setting achievable and measurable objectives. Let's break down the SMART acronym in the context of weight loss:
- **Specific**: Instead of a vague goal like "lose weight," be specific. Target a weight loss of, for example, "6 pounds in 90 days."
- **Measurable**: How will you track your progress? Daily weigh-ins (focusing on trends over daily fluctuations) and taking body measurements can be helpful.
- **Attainable**: Ensure your target weight loss is realistic and achievable within the 90-day timeframe.
- **Relevant**: Your goal should align with your overall health and well-being goals.

- **Time-bound:** Set a specific timeframe for achieving your goal, in this case, 90 days.

Example of a SMART Weight Loss Goal:
"I will lose 6 pounds in the next 90 days by tracking my daily calorie intake and participating in 30 minutes of moderate-intensity exercise most days of the week."

Breaking Down Your Goal into Smaller Steps
Setting smaller, achievable milestones throughout your 90-day program can keep you motivated and on track. Here's how to break down your overall weight loss goal:

- **Weekly Targets:** Divide your total weight loss target by the number of weeks (90 days / 7 days/week = 12.8 weeks). Aim to lose approximately 0.5-1 pound per week (round to 1 pound for simplicity).
- **Monthly Milestones:** Set mini-goals for the end of each month. For example, if you aim to lose 6 pounds in total, you could strive to lose 2 pounds by the end of month 1, 4 pounds by the end of month 2, and reach your final target by the end of month 3.

Strategies for Staying Motivated and Achieving Your Goals

- **Track Your Progress**: Regularly monitor your weight and body measurements. Seeing progress, even in small increments, can be a powerful motivator.
- **Celebrate Milestones**: Acknowledge and celebrate your achievements, big or small. This reinforces positive behaviors and keeps you motivated.
- **Find an Accountability Partner**: Enlist the support of a friend, family member, or online weight loss community for encouragement and accountability.
- **Focus on Non-Scale Victories**: Don't just focus on the scale. Celebrate non-scale victories such as increased energy levels, better fitting clothes, or improved sleep quality. These positive changes highlight the benefits of your efforts.
- **Embrace Setbacks**: Everyone encounters setbacks. Don't let them derail your progress. Acknowledge the setback, learn from it, and recommit to your goals.
- **Reward Yourself**: Set healthy rewards for reaching milestones. This could be a new

workout outfit, a relaxing massage, or an activity you enjoy.

- **Visualize Success**: Take a moment each day to visualize yourself achieving your goals. See yourself reaching your target weight, feeling energetic, and rocking a healthy lifestyle. Positive visualization can be a powerful tool for motivation.

Building Sustainable Habits for Long-Term Success

While achieving your 90-day weight loss goal is commendable, the ultimate aim is to cultivate sustainable habits for long-term success. Here are some tips:

- **Focus on Progress, Not Perfection**: Aim for progress, not perfection. There will be days when you slip up. Forgive yourself, learn from it, and get back on track.
- **Make Gradual Changes**: Drastic changes are often unsustainable. Instead, focus on implementing small, gradual changes that you can realistically maintain over time.
- **Find Activities You Enjoy**: Physical activity shouldn't feel like punishment. Explore different activities you find enjoyable,

whether it's dancing, swimming, brisk walking, or following home workout videos.

- **Fuel Your Body with Nourishing Foods:** Don't deprive yourself; focus on eating healthy, whole foods that nourish your body and keep you feeling satisfied.
- **Prioritize Sleep:** Adequate sleep is crucial for overall health and weight management. Aim for 7-8 hours of quality sleep each night.
- **Manage Stress:** Chronic stress can sabotage weight loss efforts. Find healthy stress-management techniques like yoga, meditation, or spending time in nature.

Remember: Weight loss is a journey, not a destination. By setting realistic goals, celebrating your progress, and cultivating healthy habits, you'll be well on your way to achieving sustainable success in your 90-day program and beyond. Embrace the process, focus on building a healthy lifestyle, and empower yourself to reach your full potential.

Chapter 2

Fueling Your Transformation: Effective Nutrition Strategies for Weight Loss (Without the Gym)

In your 90-day venture towards a slimmer you, making a sound and supportable eating plan is vital. This part dives into powerful sustenance systems that don't need a gym membership, engaging you to fuel your weight reduction objectives and develop a positive relationship with food.

Grasping the Force of Food

Food is something other than food; the fuel empowers your body and assumes an urgent part in weight management. By settling on informed food decisions, you can make a calorie deficiency, the center guideline behind weight reduction, and give your body the fundamental supplements it requirements to flourish.

The Significance of Calorie Equilibrium

Envision your body as a consuming heater. Food powers this heater, giving energy to day to day exercises. Calorie balance alludes to the connection between the calories you consume daily. At the point when you consume a greater number of calories, your body stores the overabundance as fat. On the other hand, when you consume a bigger number of calories than you consume, a calorie shortfall is made, prompting weight reduction.

Working out Your Calorie Needs

The initial step is to sort out your everyday calorie needs. This number addresses the base measure of energy your body expects to keep up with its ongoing weight. There are two key parts:

•	Basal Metabolic Rate (BMR): The base calories your body needs for essential capabilities like breathing and dissemination.

•	Action Level: The calories consumed day to day exercises.

A few web-based mini-computers or applications can gauge your BMR in light of variables like age, weight, level, and orientation. When you have your

BMR, consider your action level and utilize the accompanying multipliers:

•   Inactive (next to zero activity): BMR x 1.2

•   Delicately dynamic (1-3 days of activity): BMR x 1.375

•   Modestly dynamic (3-5 days): BMR x 1.55

•   Exceptionally dynamic (6-7 days): BMR x 1.725

•   Very dynamic (competitors): BMR x 1.9

Making a Manageable Calorie Shortage

Aiming for calorie shortage could appear to be enticing, yet at the same it's frequently unreasonable and counterproductive. Here is a protected and successful methodology:

1.   Start Little: Start by making a deficiency of 300-500 calories from your determined everyday necessities. This means a weight reduction of 0.5-1 pound each week, a sound and sensible objective.

2.   Track Your Calories: Food journaling or utilizing calorie-following applications assists you with remaining aware of your admission. It

features regions for changes and keeps you responsible.

Now that you comprehend calorie balance, we should investigate explicit wholesome methodologies to help your weight reduction venture!

1. Embrace Entire Food sources:

•   The Force of Nature: Focus on entire food sources like organic products, vegetables, entire grains, and lean proteins. These are supplement thick, meaning they give fundamental nutrients, minerals, and fiber while keeping you feeling more full for longer.

•   Fiber Celebration: Burden up on fiber-rich food sources like natural products, vegetables, and entire grains. Fiber advances satiety, helps assimilation, and manages glucose levels.

•   Protein Force to be reckoned with: Incorporate protein sources like chicken, fish, beans, lentils, low-fat dairy, and tofu in each feast and bite. Protein supports digestion, assists protect with muscling mass, and advances sensations of totality.

•	Solid Fats Don't Be Tricked: Don't avoid sound fats like those tracked down in avocados, nuts, seeds, and olive oil. These fats add to satiety, support supplement assimilation, and promote general wellbeing.

2. Be careful with Stowed away Calories:

•	Peruse Food Names: Become a mark understanding investigator! Focus on serving sizes, calories, and added sugars.

•	Sugar Canny: Breaking point sweet beverages, handled food sources, and sweet tidbits. These are much of the time calorie-thick and come up short on supplements. Decide on normally sweet natural products or unsweetened drinks.

•	Be careful with Subtle Sugars: Be aware of stowed away sugars hiding in apparently quality food sources like yogurt, salad dressings, and sauces.

3. Careful Eating Enchantment:

•	Dial Back and Enjoy: Practice careful eating methods like eating gradually, biting completely, and staying away from interruptions while eating.

This advances careful utilization and assists you with perceiving satiety prompts.

•   Portion Control is Critical: Utilize more modest plates and bowls to subliminally decrease portion sizes.

•   Plan Your Dinners: Arranging feasts and bites ahead of time assists you with pursuing sound decisions and stay away from incautious choices.

•   Try not to Deny Yourself: Prohibitive weight control plans are frequently unreasonable. Permit yourself periodic treats with some restraint to stay away from desires and keep a sound connection with food.

4. Hydration Legend:

•   The Force of Water: Lack of hydration can imitate cravings for food and lead to gorging. Water assumes a significant part in different physical processes, including assimilation and supplement retention. Aim for water day to day, changing in view of your action level and environment.

•   Enliven Your Water: Imbue your water with cuts of natural product, cucumber, or spices for an invigorating and delightful curve.

•   Home grown Tea Choices: Investigate unsweetened natural teas like green tea or dandelion tea for extra medical advantages and assortment.

5. Dinner Arranging and Preparing:

•   Set aside Time and Cash: Arranging and preparing dinners ahead of time forestalls undesirable somewhat late choices and sets aside your time and cash consistently.

•   Portion Control Made Simple: Pre-partitioning tidbits and dinners assists with portion control and guarantees you stay inside your calorie objectives.

•   Solid Accommodation: Having sound bites and prepared feasts promptly accessible diminishes the impulse to go after unfortunate choices when you're in a rush.

Test Dinner Plan for Weight reduction (Without the Exercise center):

Disclaimer: This is an example plan and may require changes in light of your singular necessities and inclinations. Continuously talk with a medical care professional or enrolled dietitian for customized direction.

Breakfast (around 300-400 calories):

•	Cereal with berries and a sprinkle of nuts and seeds

•	Greek yogurt with cleaved leafy foods shower of honey

•	Entire wheat toast with fried eggs and avocado cuts

Lunch (around 400-500 calories):

•	Fish salad sandwich on entire wheat bread with lettuce and tomato

•	Lentil soup with a side plate of mixed greens

•	Barbecued chicken bosom with simmered vegetables and earthy colored rice

Supper (around 500-600 calories):

•	Salmon with cooked Brussels sprouts and quinoa

- Turkey stew with a side of entire wheat saltines

- Veggie lover pan sear with tofu, vegetables, and earthy colored rice

Snacks (around 100-200 calories each):

- Apple cuts with almond spread

- Small bunch of blended nuts and dried organic product

- Carrot sticks with hummus

- Greek yogurt with a sprinkle of granola

Keep in mind: This is only an example, and you can track down unending sound recipe choices on the web or in cookbooks. The key is to zero in on entire, natural food varieties, portion control, and making a calorie shortage.

Extra Tips for Feasible Weight reduction:

- Cook More at Home: Cooking at home permits you to control fixings and part estimates.

- Track down Solid Other options: Hankering something sweet? Decide on a piece of natural product or a little square of dull chocolate rather than sweet treats.

•	Try not to Skip Feasts: Skipping dinners can upset your digestion and lead to indulging later. Go for sound snacks over the course of the day.

•	Stand by listening to Your Body: Focus on your craving and satiety prompts. Eat until you're easily full, not stuffed.

•	Partake in the Journey: Spotlight on fostering a sound connection with food and praise your advancement, huge or little.

By executing these powerful nourishment methodologies, you can change your relationship with food, make a manageable calorie shortage, and fuel your weight reduction venture without requiring a gym membership.

Remember, consistency is vital! Center around rolling out continuous improvements that you can keep up with over the long term for enduring achievement.

Balanced Eating: The Art of Portion Control and Nutrient Harmony for Weight Loss (Without the Gym)

Embarking on your 90-day weight loss journey without a gym membership requires a strategic approach to food. This subchapter delves into the power of balanced eating, highlighting the importance of portion control and nutrient harmony for sustainable weight loss.

Understanding Balanced Eating
Imagine a healthy plate divided into sections. Balanced eating involves filling those sections with a variety of nutrient-rich foods from different food groups in appropriate proportions. This ensures your body receives the essential vitamins, minerals, and fiber it needs to function optimally, while promoting satiety and supporting your weight loss goals.

The Benefits of Balanced Eating:
- **Nutrient Powerhouse:** Balanced meals provide a complete spectrum of essential nutrients, including carbohydrates, protein, healthy fats, vitamins, and minerals. This keeps your body functioning at its best and supports overall health.

- **Satiety Symphony**: Including protein, fiber, and healthy fats in your meals promotes feelings of fullness and satisfaction. This helps you avoid overeating and unhealthy snacking throughout the day.
- **Metabolism Magic**: Consuming a variety of nutrients can help optimize your metabolism, ensuring your body burns calories efficiently.
- **Sustainable Success**: Balanced eating fosters a healthy relationship with food, making weight loss sustainable and enjoyable in the long term.

The Power of Portion Control

Portion control is a crucial component of balanced eating and weight loss. It simply refers to the amount of food you consume at each meal and snack. Here's why it matters:

- **Calorie Management**: Consuming excessive portions, even of healthy foods, can lead to a calorie surplus, hindering weight loss efforts.
- **Satiety Cues**: Eating slowly and paying attention to portion sizes allows your body time to register satiety cues, preventing overeating.
- **Mindful Consumption**: Portion control promotes mindful eating, encouraging you to

savor your food and appreciate its nutritional value.

Strategies for Effective Portion Control
- **Smaller Plates and Bowls**: Opt for smaller plates and bowls. This creates the illusion of a larger portion and helps you eat less without feeling deprived.
- **Measure It Out**: Utilize measuring cups and spoons, especially during the initial stages, to become familiar with appropriate portion sizes.
- **Focus on Nutrient Density**: Prioritize nutrient-dense foods like fruits, vegetables, and whole grains. These are naturally filling and require smaller portions to feel satisfied.
- **Read Food Labels**: Pay attention to serving sizes listed on food labels. This helps you stay mindful of portion sizes, especially with pre-packaged items.
- **Slow Down and Savor**: Eat slowly and chew thoroughly. This allows your body time to register satiety cues and prevents overeating.
- **Listen to Your Body**: Stop eating when you're comfortably full, not stuffed. It

takes time for your brain to register satiety, so avoid rushing through meals.

Creating Balanced Meals on a Plate

Here's a simple approach to creating balanced meals on your plate, keeping portion control in mind:

- **Half Your Plate:** Fill half your plate with non-starchy vegetables like leafy greens, broccoli, carrots, or bell peppers. These are low in calories and high in fiber, promoting satiety and adding essential vitamins and minerals.

- **Quarter Protein Power:** Dedicate a quarter of your plate to lean protein sources like grilled chicken, fish, beans, lentils, or tofu. Protein keeps you feeling full for longer and helps preserve muscle mass.

- **Quarter Carbs:** The remaining quarter of your plate can be filled with complex carbohydrates like whole grains (brown rice, quinoa), sweet potatoes, or whole-wheat bread. These provide sustained energy but should be consumed in moderation.

- **Healthy Fats Don't Be Fooled:** Include a small portion of healthy fats like avocado slices, nuts, seeds, or a drizzle of olive oil.

Healthy fats add flavor, promote satiety, and contribute to nutrient absorption.

Remember: This is just a general guideline. You can adjust portion sizes based on your individual needs and activity level. It's always best to consult with a registered dietitian or healthcare professional for personalized guidance.

Sample Balanced Meals for Weight Loss (Without the Gym):

Breakfast (Balanced and Portion-Controlled):

- Scrambled eggs with spinach and a slice of whole-wheat toast (half plate vegetables, quarter plate protein, quarter plate carbs)
- Greek yogurt with berries and a sprinkle of granola (half plate fruit, quarter plate protein)
- Oatmeal with nuts and seeds, topped with a drizzle of honey (half plate whole grain, quarter plate healthy fats, quarter plate protein)

Lunch (Balanced and Portion-Controlled):

- Tuna salad sandwich on whole-wheat bread with lettuce and tomato (half plate vegetables, quarter plate protein, quarter plate carbs)

- Lentil soup with a side salad (half plate vegetables, quarter plate protein)
- Grilled chicken breast with roasted vegetables and brown rice (half plate vegetables, quarter plate protein, quarter plate carbs)

Dinner (Balanced and Portion-Controlled):
- Salmon with roasted Brussels sprouts and quinoa (half plate vegetables, quarter plate protein, quarter plate carbs)
- Turkey chili with a side of whole-wheat crackers (half plate vegetables, quarter plate protein, quarter plate carbs)
- Vegetarian stir-fry with tofu, vegetables, and brown rice (half plate vegetables, quarter plate protein, quarter plate carbs)

Tips for Building Balanced Meals:
- **Get Creative:** Explore a variety of healthy recipes to keep your meals interesting and prevent boredom. There are countless options online and in cookbooks for balanced and delicious meals.

- **Seasoning is Key**: Don't shy away from herbs and spices. They add flavor to your food, reducing the need for unhealthy additives like salt or sugar.
- **Leftovers are Your Friend**: Cook larger portions and save leftovers for another meal. This saves time and ensures you have healthy options readily available.
- **Plan Your Snacks**: Include healthy snacks throughout the day to prevent overeating at meals. Choose options like fruits, vegetables with hummus, nuts, or yogurt.
- **Don't Fear Fat**: Healthy fats are essential for a balanced diet. Include them in moderation as part of your meals.
- **Stay Hydrated**: Drinking plenty of water throughout the day promotes satiety and helps you make healthy food choices.

Beyond the Plate: Cultivating a Balanced Mindset

Balanced eating goes beyond just portion control and nutrient ratios. Here's how to cultivate a balanced mindset around food:

- **Focus on Progress, Not Perfection**: Aim for progress, not perfection. There will be days when you slip up. Forgive yourself, learn from it, and get back on track with your balanced eating approach.

- **Enjoy the Journey:** Develop a positive relationship with food. Savor your meals, appreciate the variety and taste, and focus on nourishing your body.
- **Listen to Your Body:** Learn to recognize your hunger and satiety cues. Eat when you're hungry and stop when you're comfortably full.
- **Don't Deprive Yourself:** Restrictive diets are often unsustainable. Allow yourself occasional treats in moderation to avoid cravings and maintain a healthy relationship with food.
- **Mindful Eating Practices:** Incorporate mindful eating practices like slowing down, putting away distractions while eating, and focusing on the taste and texture of your food.

By mastering the art of balanced eating and applying effective portion control strategies, you can create a sustainable approach to weight loss. Remember, consistency is key! Focus on making gradual changes and building a healthy relationship with food, empowering you to achieve your goals and cultivate a healthy lifestyle for the long term.

Healthy Snacking: Conquering Cravings with Nutritious and Delicious Options (Without the Gym)

Conquering cravings is a crucial battle in your 90-day weight loss journey without a gym membership. Reaching for unhealthy snacks can derail your progress. This subchapter equips you with an arsenal of delicious and nutritious snack options to curb cravings, keep you feeling satisfied, and support your weight loss goals.

Understanding the Power of Healthy Snacking: Strategic snacking can be your weight loss ally, not your enemy. Here's why:

- **Curbs Cravings:** Healthy snacks can bridge the gap between meals, preventing excessive hunger and unhealthy snack choices later.
- **Boosts Metabolism:** Small, regular snacks can help regulate blood sugar levels, preventing energy crashes and potentially boosting your metabolism.
- **Provides Essential Nutrients:** Including nutrient-rich snacks in your diet ensures

your body receives the vitamins, minerals, and fiber it needs throughout the day.
- **Promotes Satiety**: Choosing the right snacks can keep you feeling full and satisfied, reducing the urge to overeat at meals.

The Art of Choosing Healthy Snacks:
Not all snacks are created equal. Here are key principles for selecting healthy options:
- **Focus on Whole Foods**: Prioritize whole, unprocessed foods like fruits, vegetables, nuts, seeds, and yogurt. These offer a complete nutritional package and promote satiety.
- **Fiber is Your Friend**: Seek out snacks rich in fiber, which keeps you feeling fuller for longer and aids digestion. Fruits, vegetables, nuts, and whole grains are excellent sources.
- **Protein Power**: Include protein sources like nuts, yogurt, cottage cheese, or hard-boiled eggs in your snacks. Protein keeps you feeling satisfied and helps preserve muscle mass.
- **Healthy Fats Don't Be Fooled**: Don't shy away from healthy fats like those found in nuts, seeds, and avocado. They promote satiety, support nutrient absorption, and add flavor.

- **Mind the Sugar Content**: Limit sugary snacks and drinks. Opt for naturally sweet fruits or unsweetened beverages to avoid blood sugar spikes and crashes.
- **Read Food Labels**: Become a label-reading detective! Pay attention to serving sizes, calories, and added sugars to make informed choices.

Examples of Delicious and Nutritious Snacks:
Fresh and Fruity:
- Apple slices with almond butter or nut butter of your choice
- Berries with a dollop of Greek yogurt
- Pear with a sprinkle of cinnamon
- Sliced melon or pineapple
- Frozen grapes (a refreshing and healthy alternative to sugary treats)

Veggie Power:
- Carrot sticks with hummus
- Cucumber slices with a sprinkle of chili powder and lime juice
- Bell pepper slices with guacamole
- Baby carrots with a light yogurt dip
- Cherry tomatoes with a drizzle of balsamic vinegar

Nut and Seed Sensations:

- Handful of mixed nuts (almonds, cashews, walnuts)
- Trail mix made with nuts, seeds, and dried fruit (be mindful of added sugar)
- Sunflower seeds (a good source of healthy fats and vitamin E)
- Roasted chickpeas (a crunchy and protein-rich option)
- Chia seed pudding (made with chia seeds, milk, and your favorite flavorings)

Protein Powerhouse Snacks:

- Hard-boiled eggs (a classic and portable protein source)
- Greek yogurt with berries and a sprinkle of granola
- Cottage cheese with sliced vegetables
- Edamame pods (steamed or roasted)
- Turkey slices with a slice of whole-wheat bread and mustard

Additional Tips for Healthy Snacking:

- **Plan Your Snacks:** Planning out your snacks for the week helps you make healthy choices and prevents reaching for unhealthy options when hunger strikes.
- **Portion Control Matters:** Even healthy snacks can be calorie-dense. Practice portion

control and use tools like measuring cups or small containers.

- **Stay Hydrated**: Dehydration can mimic hunger pangs. Keep a reusable water bottle with you and sip on water throughout the day.
- **Don't Skip Meals**: Skipping meals can lead to overeating later. Aim for regular meals and healthy snacks throughout the day to maintain balanced blood sugar levels.
- **Listen to Your Body**: Pay attention to your hunger cues. Don't wait until you're ravenous to reach for a snack.
- **Make It Fun!**: Explore healthy recipes and experiment with different flavor combinations to keep your snacks exciting.

Curbing Specific Cravings:

- **Sweet Cravings**: Opt for naturally sweet fruits, frozen yogurt, or dark chocolate squares instead of sugary treats.
- **Salty Cravings**: Satisfy your salt cravings with air-popped popcorn seasoned with herbs or spices, roasted chickpeas, or a small handful of nuts. You can also try sliced vegetables with a light yogurt dip or a small

serving of edamame for a more balanced option.

- **Crunchy Cravings:** Reach for raw vegetables like carrots, celery, or bell peppers with hummus or a light yogurt dip. Alternatively, enjoy air-popped popcorn, roasted chickpeas, or a handful of mixed nuts for a satisfying crunch.

Preparing Healthy Snacks in Advance:
- **Save Time and Money:** Prepping healthy snacks in advance saves time throughout the week and prevents unhealthy last-minute choices.
- **Portion Control Made Easy:** Pre-portioning snacks helps you stick to your calorie goals and avoid overeating.
- **Convenience is Key:** Having healthy snacks readily available reduces the temptation to grab unhealthy options when you're short on time.

Sample Meal Prep Ideas for Healthy Snacks:
- Wash and cut fruits and vegetables like carrots, celery, and bell peppers for easy dipping.
- Prepare a batch of hard-boiled eggs for a quick and protein-rich snack.

- Whip up a batch of chia seed pudding with your favorite flavorings to enjoy throughout the week.
- Portion out individual bags of nuts, trail mix, or dried fruit to avoid overindulging.
- Roast a batch of chickpeas and season them with your favorite herbs and spices for a crunchy and protein-packed snack.

Remember: Consistency is key! By incorporating these healthy snacking strategies and delicious options into your 90-day journey, you can effectively curb cravings, stay energized throughout the day, and support your weight loss goals without requiring a gym membership. Explore different flavors and combinations to keep things interesting and create a sustainable healthy snacking routine that works for you. Happy Snacking!

Intermittent Fasting: Exploring an Alternative Eating Pattern for Weight Loss (Without the Gym)

In your 90-day weight loss journey without a gym membership, you might be curious about alternative eating patterns that can support your goals. This subchapter delves into intermittent fasting (IF), explaining how this approach can potentially aid weight loss and providing guidance for safe and effective implementation.

What is Intermittent Fasting?

Intermittent fasting (IF) is an eating pattern that cycles between periods of fasting and eating. Unlike traditional calorie restriction diets, IF focuses on *when* you eat, not necessarily *what* you eat within your eating windows. There are various IF protocols, each with different fasting and eating durations.

Popular Intermittent Fasting Protocols:

- **16/8 Method**: This involves fasting for 16 hours and restricting your eating window to 8 hours each day. This is a popular and beginner-friendly approach.
- **5:2 Diet**: Eat normally for 5 days of the week and restrict your calorie intake to 500-600 calories on 2 non-consecutive days.
- **Eat Stop Eat**: This method involves a 24-hour fast once or twice a week.

How Can Intermittent Fasting Aid Weight Loss?

While the mechanism isn't fully understood, IF may promote weight loss through several potential pathways:

- **Calorie Restriction**: By limiting your eating window, you naturally consume fewer calories overall, which can lead to weight loss.
- **Increased Insulin Sensitivity**: Fasting periods may improve your body's sensitivity to insulin, a hormone that regulates blood sugar levels. This can promote fat burning for energy.
- **Metabolic Switch**: Extended fasting periods may trigger your body to switch from burning glucose (sugar) for energy to burning stored fat reserves.

Potential Benefits of Intermittent Fasting (Beyond Weight Loss):

- **Improved Blood Sugar Control**: IF may be beneficial for individuals with prediabetes or type 2 diabetes by improving insulin sensitivity and blood sugar management.
- **Reduced Inflammation**: Studies suggest that IF may have anti-inflammatory effects, potentially reducing the risk of chronic diseases.

- **Enhanced Brain Function**: Some research suggests that IF may improve cognitive function and memory.

Important Considerations Before Trying Intermittent Fasting:

Intermittent fasting is not a one-size-fits-all approach. Here are some crucial points to consider before embarking on this eating pattern:

- **Consult Your Doctor**: It's essential to consult with your healthcare professional before starting IF, especially if you have any underlying health conditions, are pregnant, or breastfeeding.
- **Listen to Your Body**: Pay attention to your body's signals. If you experience excessive hunger, dizziness, or fatigue, adjust the protocol or discontinue IF altogether.
- **Hydration is Key**: Stay well-hydrated throughout your fasting windows by drinking plenty of water, unsweetened tea, or black coffee.
- **Nutrient-Rich Eating**: Make sure to prioritize nutrient-rich foods during your eating windows to ensure your body receives

all the essential vitamins and minerals it
needs.

- **Not a Magic Bullet**: Combine IF with a
  healthy diet and lifestyle changes for
  optimal results.

Getting Started with Intermittent Fasting:

If you decide to try IF, here are some tips for a
smooth transition:

- **Start Gradually**: Begin with shorter fasting
  windows and gradually increase the duration
  as your body adapts.
- **Choose a Protocol that Fits Your Lifestyle**:
  Select an IF protocol that aligns with your
  daily routine and preferences.
- **Focus on Healthy Eating**: During your eating
  windows, prioritize whole, unprocessed
  foods, lean proteins, healthy fats, and
  complex carbohydrates.
- **Break the Fast Wisely**: Don't overeat
  during your eating window. Break your fast
  with a balanced meal and avoid sugary or
  processed foods.
- **Listen to Your Body**: Pay attention to
  hunger cues and adjust the fasting window as

needed. Don't push yourself beyond your limits

.

Remember: Intermittent fasting is an eating pattern, not a diet. It's a potential tool to support weight loss, but it's not guaranteed to work for everyone. Always prioritize your health and consult with a healthcare professional before making significant changes to your diet.

Combining Intermittent Fasting with a Balanced Diet

Whether you choose to incorporate IF or stick with a traditional calorie-restricted diet, a balanced approach to food is crucial. Here's how to combine IF with healthy eating principles:

- **Focus on Whole Foods**: Prioritize whole, unprocessed foods like fruits, vegetables, whole grains, and lean proteins during your eating windows.
- **Protein Power**: Include protein sources like chicken, fish, beans, lentils, or tofu at every meal and snack. Protein promotes satiety and helps preserve muscle mass.
- **Healthy Fats Don't Be Fooled**: Don't shy away from healthy fats like those found in avocados, nuts, seeds, and olive oil. These

fats contribute to satiety, support nutrient absorption, and promote overall health.

- **Mindful Eating**: Practice mindful eating principles during your eating windows. Savor your food, chew thoroughly, and avoid distractions while eating.
- **Stay Hydrated**: Drink plenty of water throughout the day, especially during fasting windows, to stay hydrated and support overall health.
- **Plan Your Meals and Snacks**: Planning meals and healthy snacks for your eating windows helps you make healthy choices and avoid impulsive decisions.
- **Sample Meal Plan for Intermittent Fasting (16/8 Method):**

Disclaimer: This is a sample plan and may need adjustments based on your individual needs and preferences. Always consult with a healthcare professional or registered dietitian for personalized guidance.

Eating Window (8 Hours):

- **Breakfast (around 8:00 AM)**: Greek yogurt with berries and a sprinkle of granola, or scrambled eggs with spinach and a slice of whole-wheat toast.

- **Lunch (around 1:00 PM):** Tuna salad sandwich on whole-wheat bread with lettuce and tomato, or lentil soup with a side salad.
- **Snack (around 4:00 PM):** Handful of mixed nuts and dried fruit, or carrot sticks with hummus.
- **Dinner (around 7:00 PM):** Salmon with roasted Brussels sprouts and quinoa, or turkey chili with a side of whole-wheat crackers.

Fasting Window (16 Hours):

During this period, focus on water, unsweetened tea, or black coffee to stay hydrated.

Remember: This is just a sample, and you can adjust meal timings and portions based on your preferences and hunger cues. The key is to prioritize nutrient-rich foods and maintain a calorie deficit for weight loss.

Is Intermittent Fasting Right for You?

The decision to try intermittent fasting is a personal one. Here are some factors to consider:

- **Lifestyle**: Consider your daily routine and whether IF fits your schedule and preferences.
- **Health Conditions**: If you have any underlying health conditions, consult with your doctor before attempting IF.
- **Pregnancy and Breastfeeding**: IF is not recommended for pregnant or breastfeeding women.
- **Listen to Your Body**: Pay attention to your body's signals. If you experience negative side effects, discontinue IF and consult with a healthcare professional.

Intermittent fasting can be a valuable tool to support weight loss, but it's not a magic bullet. Focus on a balanced and sustainable approach to food, incorporate healthy lifestyle habits, and consult with a healthcare professional before making significant changes to your diet.

In conclusion, this subchapter has explored the potential benefits and considerations of intermittent fasting for weight loss. It's one approach you can explore within your 90-day journey, but remember to prioritize your health and choose a strategy that aligns with your lifestyle and preferences. By combining healthy eating habits with effective strategies like balanced meals, portion control, and potentially intermittent fasting, you can empower yourself to achieve your weight loss goals without requiring a gym membership.

Chapter 3

Unleash Your Inner Athlete - Effective Home Workouts for Weight Loss (Without the Gym)

Leaving on your 90-day weight reduction venture without a gym membership doesn't mean forfeiting a strong gym routine daily practice. In this part, we'll disclose various successful home exercises intended to shape your build, burn calories, and push you towards your weight loss objectives.

Advantages of Home Exercises:

•   Convenience is The best: Work out individually and plan, dispensing with the requirement for drives or gym membership

•   No Equipment Required: Large numbers of these activities use your own bodyweight, so no extravagant hardware is required.

•   Customized Daily practice: Design your exercises to your wellness level and objectives.

Begin slow and steadily increase power as you gain strength.

•	Protection and Solace: Work out in the security of your own home, liberated from judgment and feeling good in your own space.

Getting everything rolling with Home Exercises:

Prior to jumping into these exercises, here are a few fundamental tips:

•	Warm-Up: Consistently play out a 5-10 moment get ready to set up your body for work out. This incorporates light cardio like hopping jacks, running set up, or arm circles, trailed by unique stretches.

•	Cool-Down: Don't disregard the cool-down! Devote 5-10 minutes to static stretches to further develop adaptability and forestall muscle irritation.

•	Pay attention to Your Body: Begin slow and step by step increase power and span as you get more grounded. Try not to drive yourself to the place of agony.

•	Form Over Speed: Spotlight on appropriate form for each activity to augment results and forestall injury. If necessary, lower the intensity or number of repetitions to keep up with appropriate form

•	Hydration is Critical: Remain hydrated all through your exercise by tasting water routinely.

•	Make an Exercise Space: Assign an agreeable space in your home with adequate space to move openly and securely.

•	Track down an Exercise Mate: Spur yourself by working out with a companion or relative basically or face to face.

•	Keep tabs on Your Development: Monitoring your exercises and advance can be an incredible inspiration. Use an exercise diary or wellness application.

Test Home Exercise Timetables:

The following are two example exercise timetables to assist you with beginning. Pick a timetable that lines up with your wellness level and accessible time. Keep in mind, these are simply models, and you can change them in view of your necessities:

Plan 1: Novice (3 Exercises each Week)

- Monday: Full Body Strength Preparing (Definite later in the section)

- Wednesday: Cardio and Center Exercise (Definite later in the section)

- Friday: Dynamic Rest (Light action like strolling, yoga, or extending)

Plan 2: Middle (4-5 Exercises each Week)

- Monday: Chest area Strength Preparing (Definite later in the section)

- Tuesday: Cardio (Definite later in the section)

- Wednesday: Lower Body Strength Preparing (Definite later in the part)

- Thursday: Dynamic Rest (Light movement like strolling, yoga, or extending)

- Friday: HIIT Exercise (Definite later in the part) (Discretionary)

The Fundamental Home Exercise Activities:

Presently, we should dig into the particular activities you can integrate into your home exercises. These activities target different muscle gatherings and can be consolidated to make powerful schedules.

Warm-Up:

•	Bouncing Jacks: 3 arrangements of 30 seconds

•	High Knees: 3 arrangements of 30 seconds

•	Butt Kicks: 3 arrangements of 30 seconds

•	Arm Circles (forward and in reverse): 3 arrangements of 10 repetitions every bearing

•	Shoulder Continues (forward and in reverse): 3 arrangements of 10 repetitions every bearing

Strength Preparing:

Full Body Strength Preparing:

•	Squats: Focus on your quads, hamstrings, and glutes. Perform 3 arrangements of 10-15 repetitions with appropriate structure.

•	Jumps: Work your quads, glutes, and center. Complete 3 arrangements of 10-12 repetition for every leg.

•	Push-Ups: Changed renditions on knees or against a wall are perfect for novices. Aim however, for many reiterations as could be expected under the circumstances with appropriate structure.

•	Columns: Use furniture or opposition groups for lines that focus on your back muscles. Perform 3 arrangements of 10-12 repetitions.

•	Board: This isometric activity draws in your center, back, and shoulders. Hold a board for 3 arrangements of 30-60 seconds each.

Chest area Strength Preparing:

•	Push-Ups (as portrayed above) or Push-Up Varieties: Precious stone push-ups (hands near one another) focus on your rear arm muscles all the more with great intensity. Perform 3 arrangements of however many repetitions as could reasonably be expected with appropriate structure.

•	Above Press: Use water bottles or canned products for an above press that reinforces your shoulders. Complete 3 arrangements of 10-12 repetitions.

- Bicep Twists: Improve bicep strength with bodyweight twists or ad libbed loads like water bottles. Hold back nothing of 10-12 repetitions.

- Rear arm muscle Plunges: Use a solid seat for rear arm muscle plunges that focus on the rear of your upper arms. Perform 3 arrangements of whatever number repetitions as could be expected under the circumstances with appropriate structure.

Lower Body Strength Preparing:

- Squats (as depicted above): You can add varieties like leap squats or single-leg squats as you progress.

- Lurches (as depicted above): Take a stab at strolling rushes or opposite jumps for added challenge.

- Step-Ups: Track down a durable seat or step and perform step-ups to fortify your quads and glutes. Complete 3 arrangements of 10-12 repetitions for every leg.

- Glute Scaffolds: Actuate your glutes with glute spans, lying on your back with knees twisted and raising your hips off the ground. Perform 3 arrangements of 10-15 repetitions.

• Calf Raises: Stand on the bundles of your feet and raise your impact points over and over to focus on your calves. Complete 3 arrangements of 15-20 repetitions.

Center Preparation:

• Board (as portrayed above): Intend to increase hold time as you get more grounded.

• Crunches: Focus on your upper abs with crunches. Perform 3 arrangements of 15-20 repetitions.

• Russian Turns: Draw in your obliques with Russian turns, pivoting your middle from one side to another while lying on your back with knees twisted and feet level on the floor. Complete 3 arrangements of 10-12 repetitions for each side.

• Side Board: Reinforce your obliques with side boards, standing firm on your body in a board footing on each side in turn. Hold back nothing of 30-60 seconds each side.

Cardio Exercises:

•	Bouncing Jacks: A straightforward and viable cardio work out. Complete 3 arrangements of 30-60 seconds.

•	High Knees: Run set up while bringing your knees high towards your chest. Perform 3 arrangements of 30-60 seconds.

•	Butt Kicks: Run set up while kicking your heels towards your glutes. Complete 3 arrangements of 30-60 seconds.

•	Hopping Jacks with Squats: Consolidate bouncing jacks with a squat at the lower part of each leap for an additional test. Perform 3 arrangements of 30-60 seconds.

•	Burpees: This full-body practice gets your pulse up and works different muscle gatherings. Begin in a squat position, hop back to a board, play out a push-up, bounce your feet back to hunch down, and afterward hop up dangerously. Aim for many repetitions as would be prudent with appropriate structure.

•	Step Climbing: Assuming you have steps in your home, use them for step climbing stretches.

- • Running Set up: A basic yet viable method for hoisting your pulse. Keep a moderate to extreme focus for 3 arrangements of 30-60 seconds.

HIIT (Intense cardio exercise) Exercise:

HIIT exercises include substituting short explosions of serious activity with times of rest or low-power movement. This kind of preparing consumes calories effectively and supports your digestion.

Test HIIT Exercise:

- • Warm-Up (as portrayed over): 5 minutes

- • High Knees: 30 seconds at extreme focus

- • Rest: 30 seconds

- • Bouncing Jacks: 30 seconds at extreme focus

- • Rest: 30 seconds

- • Squats: 30 seconds at focused energy

- • Rest: 30 seconds

- • Burpees: 30 seconds at focused energy (change if necessary)

- Rest: 30 seconds

- Rehash this circuit 3-4 times

- Cool-Down (as depicted over): 5 minutes

Cool-Down:

- Static Stretches: Hold each stretch for 30-60 seconds. Center around significant muscle bunches worked during your exercise.

Keep in mind: These are simply test exercises. Change them in light of your wellness level, inclinations, and accessible hardware. There are innumerable varieties and movements for these activities, so investigate and find what turns out best for you.

Movement Tips:

- Increase Reps or Sets: As you get more grounded, progressively increase the quantity of repetitions or sets you perform for each activity.

- Decrease Rest Periods: Decrease your rest time between sets as your perseverance moves along.

- Add Weight: Once bodyweight practices become excessively simple, consider adding weight with obstruction groups, water bottles, or filled rucksacks.

• Increase Force: Pick additional difficult varieties of activities as you progress.

Additional Resources:

• Online Wellness Resources: Various web-based stages offer free or membership based exercise recordings and schedules. Investigate these resources for motivation and direction.

• Portable Wellness Applications: Numerous wellness applications can assist you with following exercises, give customized schedules, and deal informative recordings for legitimate structure.

Remaining Spurred:

Remaining spurred all through your 90-day venture is critical. Here are a few hints to move you along:

• Put forth Brilliant Objectives: Set Explicit, Quantifiable, Feasible, Significant, and Time-Bound objectives to keep tabs on your development and celebrate achievements.

- •   Track down an Exercise Mate: Working out with a companion or relative can expand responsibility and make practice more pleasant.

- •   Reward Yourself: Praise your accomplishments and achievements with sound prizes, not food-related ones.

- •   Keep tabs on Your Development: Keeping an exercise diary or utilizing a wellness application permits you to screen your advancement and picture your improvement.

- •   Pay attention to Peppy Music: Playful music can empower you during your exercises.

- •   Center around the Good: Celebrate how your body feels more grounded and more invigorated as you progress.

- •   Find Exercises You Appreciate: Pick exercise styles you see as tomfoolery and locking in. Practice shouldn't feel like an errand.

Safety Considerations:

- • **Listen to Your Body:** Don't push yourself to the point of pain. Take rest days when needed and avoid overtraining.

- **Maintain Proper Form**: Always prioritize proper form over speed or weight. Incorrect form can lead to injury.
- **Consult a Healthcare Professional**: If you have any underlying health conditions, consult with a healthcare professional before starting a new exercise routine.

The Takeaway:

By incorporating these home workouts into your 90-day weight loss journey, you can achieve significant results without a gym membership. Remember, consistency is key! Stick to your workout routine, track your progress, and celebrate your achievements.

Embrace the journey of becoming your own home gym warrior. You have the power to unlock your inner athlete and transform your physique, all within the comfort of your own space.

This chapter has equipped you with the knowledge and resources to embark on effective home workouts. Remember, consistency, proper form, and finding a workout style you enjoy are key ingredients for success. Now go forth and unleash your inner athlete!

Bodyweight Exercises: Master Effective Bodyweight Exercises for Strength and Toning

Building strength and muscle tone doesn't require a fancy gym membership. In fact, some of the most effective exercises use nothing but your own body weight! This subchapter will guide you through a variety of bodyweight exercises designed to target different muscle groups and help you achieve your weight loss and toning goals in 90 days, all from the comfort of your own home.

Benefits of Bodyweight Exercises:

- **Convenience:** No gym membership or equipment needed. You can do these exercises anywhere, anytime.
- **Versatility:** A wide range of exercises can target all major muscle groups.
- **Improves Functional Fitness:** Bodyweight exercises mimic everyday movements, improving overall strength and balance for daily activities.

- **Reduced Risk of Injury**: Bodyweight exercises are low-impact, making them suitable for beginners and those with joint issues.
- **Boosts Metabolism**: Building muscle increases your resting metabolic rate, helping you burn more calories even at rest.

Getting Started with Bodyweight Exercises:
- **Warm-up**: Before starting your workout, spend 5-10 minutes warming up with light cardio (jumping jacks, jumping rope) and dynamic stretches (arm circles, leg swings) to prepare your muscles for exercise and prevent injury.
- **Form Matters**: Focus on proper form for each exercise. This will maximize results and minimize the risk of injury.
- **Progression**: As you get stronger, increase the difficulty of the exercises by adding variations, increasing repetitions, or decreasing rest periods.
- **Listen to Your Body**: Rest when needed and don't push yourself through pain.

Sample Bodyweight Workout Routines:

Here are two sample bodyweight routines designed to target your entire body. You can perform these routines 2-3 times per week with at least one rest day in between.

Routine 1 (Upper Body Focus):
1. Push-ups (modified on knees if needed): 3 sets of 10-12 repetitions.
2. Dips (using a chair or bench): 3 sets of 10-12 repetitions.
3. Plank: 3 sets of 30-60 seconds hold.
4. Wall Sits: 3 sets of 30-60 seconds hold.
5. Inverted Rows (using a sturdy table or bar): 3 sets of 10-12 repetitions.
6. Superman: 3 sets of 10-12 repetitions per side.

Routine 2 (Lower Body Focus):
1. Squats: 3 sets of 12-15 repetitions.
2. Lunges (alternating legs): 3 sets of 10-12 repetitions per leg.
3. Glute Bridges: 3 sets of 12-15 repetitions.
4. Side Lunges: 3 sets of 10-12 repetitions per leg.
5. Calf Raises: 3 sets of 15-20 repetitions.
6. Mountain Climbers: 3 sets of 30 seconds work, 30 seconds rest.

Detailed Exercise Descriptions:
Upper Body:
- **Push-ups:** A classic bodyweight exercise targeting your chest, triceps, and shoulders. Start in a high plank position with hands shoulder-width apart. Lower your chest towards the ground while keeping your core engaged and back straight. Push back up to the starting position. Modify on your knees if needed.
- **Dips:** Strengthens your triceps and shoulders. Sit on a sturdy chair or bench with your hands gripping the edge beside your hips. Lower yourself down until your elbows bend at a 90-degree angle. Push back up to the starting position.
- **Plank:** Engages your core and shoulders. Start in a push-up position with your forearms on the ground. Keep your body in a straight line from head to heels, engaging your core muscles.
- **Wall Sits:** Targets your quads and core. Stand with your back against a wall and slowly slide down until your knees are bent at a 90-degree angle. Hold this position for the designated time.

- **Inverted Rows**: Strengthens your back and biceps. Find a sturdy table or bar at waist height. Grip the bar with an overhand grip and hang with your arms straight. Row yourself up until your chest nearly touches the bar. Lower yourself back down with control.
- **Superman**: Works your lower back and glutes. Lie on your stomach with your arms and legs extended. Lift your chest, arms, and legs slightly off the ground, hold for a second, then lower back down.

Lower Body:
- **Squats**: A fundamental exercise targeting your quads, glutes, and hamstrings. Stand with your feet shoulder-width apart, toes slightly pointed outwards. Lower yourself down as if sitting in a chair, keeping your back straight and core engaged. Descend until your thighs are parallel to the ground (or as low as comfortable), then push back up to the starting position.
- **Lunges**: Strengthens your quads, glutes, and hamstrings while improving balance. Step forward with one leg, lowering your body until both knees are bent at 90-degree

angles. Ensure your front knee tracks over your ankle and your back knee doesn't touch the ground. Push back up to the starting position and repeat with the other leg.

- **Glute Bridges:** Isolates your glutes for a toned backside. Lie on your back with knees bent and feet flat on the floor. Lift your hips off the ground until your body forms a straight line from shoulders to knees. Squeeze your glutes at the top, then slowly lower back down.

- **Side Lunges:** Targets your inner and outer thighs while improving hip stability. Stand with your feet hip-width apart. Step out to the side with one leg, lowering your hips until your knee bends at a 90-degree angle. Keep your other leg straight. Push back up to the starting position and repeat with the other leg.

- **Calf Raises:** Strengthens your calves for better stability and posture. Stand with your feet shoulder-width apart and rise up onto your toes. Hold for a second at the top, then lower your heels back down. You can perform this exercise on a step or curb to increase difficulty.

- **Mountain Climbers**: A dynamic exercise that works your core, legs, and shoulders. Start in a high plank position. Bring one knee towards your chest in a running motion, then switch legs quickly. Maintain a fast pace for the designated work period.

Core:

- **Plank Variations**: The plank can be modified in various ways to target different core muscles. Try side planks (holding a plank on one side with your hips stacked), hollow body holds (lying on your back with your lower back pressed into the ground and arms and legs raised), or plank variations with arm or leg extensions for an extra challenge.
- **Crunches**: A classic core exercise that targets your upper abs. Lie on your back with knees bent and feet flat on the floor. Engage your core and lift your upper back off the ground, bringing your chest towards your knees. Lower back down with control and repeat.
- **Russian Twists**: Works your obliques for a defined midsection. Sit on the floor with your knees bent and feet flat. Lean back slightly with your core engaged and twist

your torso from side to side, bringing your hands towards the ground on each side.

Additional Tips:

- **Increase Intensity**: As you get stronger, increase the difficulty of these exercises by adding variations, increasing repetitions/sets, or decreasing rest periods.
- **Focus on Form**: Proper form is crucial for maximizing results and preventing injury. Don't sacrifice form for heavier weight or more repetitions.
- **Combine with Cardio**: Bodyweight exercises are great for building strength and toning, but don't forget about cardio! Aim for at least 150 minutes of moderate-intensity cardio per week to boost your weight loss efforts.
- **Listen to Your Body**: Take rest days when needed and don't push yourself through pain.

Remember, consistency is key! Sticking to a regular workout routine with proper form and progressive overload will help you achieve your weight loss and toning goals in 90 days. By utilizing these bodyweight exercises, you can build strength, improve your overall fitness, and sculpt a toned physique without ever stepping foot in a gym.

HIIT (High-Intensity Interval Training): Create a Home HIIT Routine

High-Intensity Interval Training (HIIT) has become a popular fitness trend for good reason. This high-intensity, short-duration workout burns serious calories, boosts metabolism, and improves cardiovascular health – all in a fraction of the time compared to traditional cardio sessions.

The beauty of HIIT? You can easily perform it at home with minimal to no equipment. This subchapter will guide you through the benefits of HIIT, provide tips for creating your own home HIIT routine, and offer sample workouts to get you started on your weight loss journey in just 90 days.

Benefits of HIIT for Weight Loss:
- **Increased Calorie Burn:** HIIT alternates between short bursts of intense activity and recovery periods. This keeps your body burning calories at an elevated rate even after your workout is finished (known as the afterburn effect).

- **Improved Efficiency**: HIIT workouts are generally shorter than traditional cardio, making them a time-efficient way to maximize your fitness results.
- **Boosts Metabolism**: The intensity of HIIT workouts helps to increase your resting metabolic rate (RMR), meaning you burn more calories even at rest.
- **Improves Cardiovascular Health**: HIIT strengthens your heart and improves your body's ability to use oxygen, leading to better overall fitness.
- **Builds Muscle**: HIIT can help to build lean muscle mass, which further increases calorie burn and improves body composition.

Creating Your Home HIIT Routine:

Here are some key things to consider when designing your home HIIT routine:

- **Warm-up**: Before jumping into high-intensity work, spend 5-10 minutes warming up with light cardio (jumping jacks, jogging in place) and dynamic stretches to prepare your muscles and joints.
- **Intensity**: During the work intervals, aim for an intensity level of 8-10 on a perceived

exertion scale (1 being easy, 10 being extremely hard). You should be working hard enough to feel breathless and unable to carry on a conversation.

- **Rest Periods**: Rest periods should be sufficient to allow you to recover enough to go all-out during the next work interval. A good starting point is a 1:2 work-to-rest ratio (30 seconds work, 60 seconds rest). As you get fitter, you can shorten your rest periods.
- **Duration**: Aim for a total workout time of 15-30 minutes. You can adjust this based on your fitness level and time constraints.
- **Frequency**: Perform HIIT workouts 2-3 times per week with at least one rest day in between to allow your body to recover.

Choosing Exercises:

The beauty of HIIT is that you can incorporate a variety of bodyweight exercises or exercises using minimal equipment. Here are some exercise ideas to get you started:

Bodyweight Exercises:
- Jumping Jacks

- High Knees
- Mountain Climbers
- Burpees
- Squat Jumps
- Lunges
- Push-ups (modified on knees if needed)
- Dips (using a chair or bench)
- Plank variations
- Crunches
- Russian Twists

Exercises with Minimal Equipment:
- Jump Rope (increases cardio intensity)
- Dumbbell exercises (squats, rows, lunges, overhead press)
- Kettlebell Swings
- Box Jumps (using a sturdy step or bench)

Sample Home HIIT Workouts:

Here are two sample HIIT workouts designed for different fitness levels. Modify the exercises or rest periods as needed to suit your abilities.

Beginner HIIT Workout:

Warm-up: 5 minutes of light cardio and dynamic stretches

Circuit 1 (Repeat 3 times with 60 seconds rest between circuits)

- Jumping Jacks: 30 seconds work
- High Knees: 30 seconds work
- Rest: 60 seconds

Circuit 2 (Repeat 3 times with 60 seconds rest between circuits)

- Squats: 30 seconds work
- Lunges (alternating legs): 30 seconds work (15 seconds per leg)
- Rest: 60 seconds

Circuit 3 (Repeat 3 times with 60 seconds rest between circuits)

- Plank: 30 seconds work
- Crunches: 30 seconds work
- Rest: 60 seconds

Cool-down: 5 minutes of light cardio and static stretches

Advanced HIIT Workout:

Warm-up: 5 minutes of light cardio and dynamic stretches

Circuit 1 (Repeat 4 times with 45 seconds rest between circuits)

- Burpees: 30 seconds work
- Mountain Climbers: 30 seconds work
- Rest: 45 seconds

Circuit 2 (Repeat 4 times with 45 seconds rest between circuits)

- Dumbbell Squats (10 reps per leg): 30 seconds work
- Dumbbell Rows (10 reps per arm): 30 seconds work
- Rest: 45 seconds

Circuit 3 (Repeat 4 times with 45 seconds rest between circuits)

- Jump Rope: 45 seconds work
- Push-ups (modified on knees if needed): 30 seconds work
- Rest: 45 seconds

Cool-down: 5 minutes of light cardio and static stretches

Progression:

As you get fitter, there are several ways to progress your HIIT workouts:

- **Increase Intensity**: Gradually increase the intensity of your work intervals by pushing yourself a little harder each time.
- **Shorten Rest Periods**: As your fitness improves, you can shorten your rest periods to increase the overall challenge of the workout.
- **Increase Work Time**: Once you're comfortable with the basic format, consider extending the work intervals or adding additional rounds to your circuits.
- **Incorporate More Challenging Exercises**: As you get stronger, try incorporating more challenging exercises like box jumps, kettlebell swings, or jump rope variations.

Safety Tips for HIIT:
- **Listen to Your Body**: HIIT is a demanding workout, so it's crucial to listen to your body. Take rest days when needed and don't push yourself through pain.
- **Proper Form**: Maintaining proper form during exercises is essential to prevent injury. If you're unsure about an exercise, don't hesitate to modify it or leave it out.

- **Start Slow:** If you're new to HIIT, it's important to start gradually and gradually increase the intensity and duration of your workouts.
- **Hydration:** Drink plenty of water before, during, and after your HIIT workouts to stay hydrated.
- **Consult a Doctor:** If you have any pre-existing health conditions, consult with your doctor before starting a HIIT program.

Remember, consistency is key! By incorporating HIIT workouts into your routine 2-3 times per week and combining them with a healthy diet, you can see significant results in your weight loss and overall fitness journey within 90 days. HIIT provides a time-efficient and effective way to burn calories, boost metabolism, and get fit in the comfort of your own home. So lace up your sneakers, put on some motivating music, and get ready to sweat!

Yoga and Pilates: Learn About Low-Impact Workouts for Flexibility and Muscle Endurance

Looking to improve your flexibility, build core strength, and achieve a toned physique without the high impact of traditional exercise? Look no further than yoga and Pilates! These mind-body practices offer a unique blend of physical postures, breathing exercises, and mindfulness that can benefit your weight loss journey in several ways.

Benefits of Yoga and Pilates for Weight Loss:
- **Improved Flexibility:** Yoga and Pilates emphasize stretching and mobility exercises, which can improve your range of motion and make everyday activities easier. Increased flexibility can also enhance your performance in other workouts.
- **Builds Core Strength:** Both yoga and Pilates focus on engaging your core muscles throughout the movements. This strengthens your abdominal and back muscles, leading to better posture, improved balance, and a more sculpted midsection.
- **Increased Mind-Body Connection:** Yoga and Pilates incorporate mindfulness and breathwork, promoting a sense of well-being and reducing stress. Stress can often lead to unhealthy eating habits, so managing stress through these practices can positively impact your weight loss efforts.

- **Low-Impact Exercise**: Yoga and Pilates are gentle on your joints, making them perfect for beginners or those with joint issues. These exercises can be a great way to stay active and burn calories without the risk of injury.
- **Improves Body Composition**: While not the primary focus, yoga and Pilates can help build lean muscle mass, which can slightly increase your resting metabolic rate and help you burn more calories at rest.

Understanding Yoga:

Yoga is an ancient practice originating in India that combines physical postures (asanas), breathing exercises (pranayama), and meditation to promote physical and mental well-being. There are many different styles of yoga, each with its own focus and intensity level. Some popular styles for weight loss and toning include:

- **Vinyasa Yoga**: A dynamic style that flows from one pose to the next, creating a more cardio-focused workout.
- **Hatha Yoga**: A gentle introduction to yoga, focusing on basic postures and proper breathing techniques.

- **Power Yoga:** A vigorous style that builds strength and endurance through challenging poses and sequences.
- **Iyengar Yoga:** Emphasizes precise alignment and the use of props to support the body in postures, making it accessible to all levels.

Understanding Pilates:

Pilates is a system of exercises developed by Joseph Pilates in the early 20th century. Pilates focuses on strengthening your core muscles, improving posture, and increasing flexibility. Pilates exercises are typically performed on a mat or using specialized equipment like reformers and chairs.

Getting Started with Yoga and Pilates:
- **Find a Class or Online Instruction:** Look for beginner-friendly yoga or Pilates classes in your area or online. There are numerous online resources offering free or paid classes for all levels.
- **Invest in a Yoga Mat:** A comfortable yoga mat will provide cushioning and support during your practice.

- **Wear Comfortable Clothing:** Choose loose-fitting clothing that allows for freedom of movement.
- **Listen to Your Body:** Don't push yourself beyond your limits. Yoga and Pilates are not about attaining perfect form but about finding modifications that work for your body.
- **Focus on Breathwork:** Proper breathing is an essential part of both yoga and Pilates. Pay attention to your breath as you move through the exercises.

Sample Yoga and Pilates Routines:

Here are some sample routines to get you started with yoga and Pilates for weight loss:

Yoga Routine (Vinyasa Flow):
- **Sun Salutations (3 rounds):** Flow through a series of poses that warm up your entire body and increase circulation.
- **Downward-Facing Dog (Adho Mukha Svanasana):** Hold for 5 breaths, stretching your hamstrings, calves, and spine.
- **Warrior II (Virabhadrasana II):** Hold for 5 breaths per side, strengthening your legs and core.

- **Triangle Pose (Trikonasana):** Hold for 5 breaths per side, opening your hips and improving flexibility.
- **Crescent Moon Pose (Anjaneyasana):** Hold for 5 breaths per side, stretching your quadriceps and lungs.
- **Plank Pose (Chaturanga Dandasana):** Hold for as long as comfortable, strengthening your core and shoulders.
- **Cobra Pose (भुजंगासन Bhujangasana):** Hold for 5 breaths, stretching your back and chest.
- **Child's Pose (Balasana):** Rest for several breaths, allowing your body to relax and recover.

Repeat this sequence 2-3 times, or adjust the poses and repetitions based on your fitness level.

Pilates Routine (Mat-Based):

- **Pelvic Tilts (continued):** Lie on your back with knees bent and feet flat on the floor. Engage your core muscles and press your lower back into the mat as you tilt your pelvis upwards. Hold for a few seconds, then slowly release and repeat 10-12 times.
- **Bridge:** Lie on your back with knees bent and feet flat on the floor. Lift your hips off the

ground until your body forms a straight line from shoulders to knees. Squeeze your glutes at the top, then slowly lower back down. Repeat 10-12 times.

- **Single Leg Circles**: Lie on your back with one leg extended and the other bent with your foot flat on the floor. Lift your extended leg a few inches off the ground and slowly make small circles with your foot, keeping your core engaged. Complete 10 circles in each direction, then switch legs and repeat.
- **Plank**: Start in a push-up position with your forearms on the ground. Keep your body in a straight line from head to heels, engaging your core muscles. Hold for 30-60 seconds, or as long as comfortable.
- **Side Plank**: Lie on your side with your forearm on the ground and your body stacked in a straight line. Lift your hips off the ground, engaging your core. Hold for 30-60 seconds per side.
- **Cat-Cow**: Start on your hands and knees with a flat back. As you inhale, arch your back and look up (cow pose). As you exhale, round your back and tuck your chin to your chest (cat pose). Repeat 10 times.

- **Roll Down**: Sit with your legs extended and reach for your toes, keeping your back straight. Slowly roll down your spine, vertebra by vertebra, until you reach your head to your knees or as far as comfortable. Hold for a few breaths, then slowly roll back up one vertebra at a time. Repeat 5-10 times.

Remember:
- Modify exercises as needed.
- Focus on proper form over speed or difficulty.
- Breathe deeply throughout the routine.

Combining Yoga and Pilates with Other Exercises:

While yoga and Pilates are excellent for building flexibility, core strength, and overall well-being, they may not be sufficient for significant weight loss on their own. Consider incorporating them with other weight loss strategies such as:

- **Healthy Diet**: Focus on eating a balanced diet rich in whole foods, fruits, vegetables, and lean protein.
- **Cardio**: Aim for at least 150 minutes of moderate-intensity cardio per week, such as

brisk walking, swimming, or cycling, to boost calorie burning.

- **Strength Training:** Building muscle mass can increase your resting metabolic rate and help you burn more calories at rest. Consider adding bodyweight exercises or light weight training to your routine.

By combining yoga and Pilates with a healthy diet and other forms of exercise, you can create a well-rounded weight loss plan that addresses multiple aspects of your health and fitness.

Remember, consistency is key! Stick to your routine for 90 days and witness the positive changes in your body and mind.

Chapter 4

Mindset and Motivation: Fueling Your 90-Day Weight Loss Journey

Losing weight requires more than just physical activity and a healthy diet. A strong mindset and unwavering motivation are crucial ingredients for success in your 90-day weight loss journey. This chapter will guide you through developing a positive mindset, overcoming challenges, and staying motivated to reach your goals.

Shifting Your Mindset:

The first step to weight loss success is shifting your mindset from one of deprivation or punishment to one of empowerment and self-care. Here are some key aspects to consider:

- **Focus on Health, Not Just Weight:** Instead of solely focusing on the number on the scale, shift your focus to improving your overall health and well-being. This includes increased energy, improved sleep, and a stronger body.
- **Embrace the Journey:** View your weight loss journey as a positive transformation, not a quick fix. Celebrate your non-scale victories like increased strength, better posture, and improved mood.
- **Develop a Growth Mindset:** Believe that you have the ability to learn, grow, and achieve your goals. Embrace challenges as opportunities to learn and adjust your approach.
- **Practice Self-Compassion:** Be kind and understanding with yourself. There will be setbacks and slip-ups along the way. Forgive yourself, learn from the experience, and get back on track.

Setting SMART Goals:

Setting clear and achievable goals is essential for staying motivated. Here's how to create SMART goals for your weight loss journey:

- **Specific**: Define your goals clearly. Instead of saying "I want to lose weight," set a specific target like "I want to lose 10 pounds in 90 days."
- **Measurable**: Track your progress towards your goals. This could be through weight loss, body measurements, or how your clothes fit.
- **Attainable**: Set realistic and achievable goals. Don't aim for unrealistic weight loss in a short period.
- **Relevant**: Choose goals that are aligned with your overall health and fitness aspirations.
- **Time-Bound**: Set a deadline for achieving your goals to stay focused and motivated.

Building Positive Habits:

Sustainable weight loss is all about creating positive lifestyle changes. Here are some tips for building healthy habits that stick:

- **Start Small**: Don't try to overhaul your entire life all at once. Begin with small, manageable changes, like incorporating one healthy meal per day or adding a short walk to your routine.

- **Focus on Progress, Not Perfection**: Aim for progress, not perfection. There will be days when you stumble. The key is to get back on track and keep moving forward.
- **Make it Enjoyable**: Choose healthy habits that you find enjoyable. Explore different exercise routines, healthy recipes, and find activities that make you feel good.
- **Accountability**: Tell a friend or family member about your goals and ask for their support. Consider joining an online weight loss community for motivation and accountability.

Strategies for Overcoming Challenges:

You will inevitably encounter challenges on your weight loss journey. Here are some strategies to help you overcome them:

- **Identify Your Triggers**: Recognize situations or emotions that tempt you to stray from your healthy habits. Develop coping mechanisms like taking a walk or practicing relaxation techniques when you encounter these triggers.

- **Plan for Obstacles:** Anticipate potential setbacks and have a plan in place to deal with them. For example, if you know you'll be attending a social event with unhealthy food choices, plan healthy snacks beforehand.
- **Positive Self-Talk:** Challenge negative thoughts with positive affirmations. Remind yourself of your goals and the progress you've made.
- **Seek Support:** Don't be afraid to ask for help from friends, family, or a therapist. Having a support system can make a big difference in staying motivated.

Staying Motivated:

Motivation is key to sticking with your weight loss plan. Here are some tips to stay motivated throughout your 90-day journey:

- **Visualize Success:** Imagine yourself achieving your goals. Create a vision board with images of your ideal physique or healthy lifestyle.
- **Reward Yourself:** Celebrate your milestones with non-food rewards like a new outfit, a massage, or a fun activity.

- **Track Your Progress**: Seeing your progress is a powerful motivator. Regularly track your weight, measurements, or how your clothes are fitting.
- **Find Inspiration**: Surround yourself with positive influences. Follow fitness blogs, read inspirational stories, or find a workout buddy to keep you accountable.
- **Focus on the Positive**: Instead of focusing on what you're giving up, focus on the positive changes you're making and how you feel better physically and mentally.
- **Practice Gratitude**: Take time each day to appreciate your body and the progress you've made. Gratitude fosters a positive outlook and keeps you motivated.
- **Make it Fun**: Choose activities you enjoy. Explore new workout routines, try healthy recipes, or find ways to make exercise and healthy eating fun.

Mindfulness and Stress Management:

Stress can be a major obstacle to weight loss. When stressed, our bodies release cortisol, a hormone that can promote weight gain. Here are some tips for managing stress and promoting mindfulness:

- **Meditation:** Regular meditation practice can help reduce stress, improve focus, and promote emotional well-being. There are many guided meditations available online or through apps to help you get started.
- **Deep Breathing Exercises:** Taking slow, deep breaths can activate the relaxation response in your body, counteracting the effects of stress.
- **Mindful Eating:** Practice mindful eating by paying attention to your body's hunger and fullness cues. Eat slowly and savor your food, avoiding distractions like television or phones.
- **Get Enough Sleep:** Aim for 7-8 hours of quality sleep each night. Sleep deprivation can disrupt hormones that regulate appetite and metabolism, making weight loss more challenging.

Remember: Weight loss is a journey, not a destination. There will be ups and downs along the way. By developing a positive mindset, setting achievable goals, and creating sustainable habits, you can fuel your motivation and achieve lasting weight loss success in 90 days and beyond. This journey is about creating a healthier, happier you, and every step you take is a step in the right direction.

Bonus Tips:

- **Find a Workout Buddy:** Having a workout partner can help you stay accountable and make exercise more enjoyable.
- **Invest in a Fitness Tracker:** Wearing a fitness tracker can help you track your steps, calories burned, and activity levels, keeping you motivated and informed.
- **Meal Prep:** Dedicate some time each week to prepping healthy meals and snacks. This will help you avoid unhealthy choices when you're short on time.
- **Drink Plenty of Water:** Staying hydrated is essential for overall health and can also help curb cravings. Aim for 8 glasses of water per day.
- **Don't Compare Yourself to Others:** Everyone's body and weight loss journey is unique. Focus on your own progress and celebrate your achievements.

By incorporating these strategies and cultivating a positive mindset, you can transform your weight loss journey into a rewarding and empowering experience. Remember, you are capable of achieving your goals and creating a healthier, happier you. Now go out there and conquer your 90 days!

Mindful Eating: Cultivate Awareness Around Food Choices for Lasting Weight Loss

In today's fast-paced world, we often eat on autopilot, mindlessly consuming food without truly registering what we're putting into our bodies. This can lead to overeating, unhealthy choices, and ultimately hinder weight loss efforts. Mindful eating, however, offers a powerful tool to transform your relationship with food and achieve lasting weight loss success in your 90-day journey.

What is Mindful Eating?

Mindful eating is the practice of paying close attention to the physical and emotional sensations associated with food. It involves bringing awareness to your thoughts, feelings, and bodily cues throughout the entire eating experience – from the moment you sit down to the moment you feel satisfied. By cultivating this awareness, you can make conscious choices about what you eat, how much you eat, and why you eat.

Benefits of Mindful Eating for Weight Loss:

- **Reduced Cravings**: Mindful eating helps you identify and manage emotional triggers for unhealthy cravings. By tuning into your body's true hunger signals, you can avoid mindless snacking and emotional eating.
- **Portion Control**: When you eat mindfully, you savor each bite and pay attention to your body's fullness cues. This can help you naturally eat less and avoid overeating.
- **Improved Digestion**: Eating slowly and chewing thoroughly allows your body to break down food more efficiently, leading to better digestion and nutrient absorption.
- **Increased Enjoyment**: Mindful eating allows you to appreciate the taste, texture, and aroma of your food, leading to a more fulfilling and enjoyable eating experience.
- **Reduced Stress**: By focusing on the present moment and your body's sensations, mindful eating can help reduce stress levels, which can positively impact your weight loss efforts.

Developing Your Mindful Eating Practice:

Here are some key practices to incorporate into your daily routine to cultivate mindful eating:

- **Create a Calm Environment**: Find a quiet, distraction-free space to enjoy your meals. Turn off the television, put away your phone, and avoid multitasking while eating.
- **Start with Gratitude**: Before taking the first bite, take a moment to appreciate your food. Consider the effort it took to bring the food to your table, be it growing, raising, preparing, or purchasing.
- **Engage Your Senses**: Pay attention to the colors, textures, and aromas of your food. Savor each bite, noticing the different flavors and sensations.
- **Chew Thoroughly**: Chewing your food thoroughly allows for better digestion and helps you feel fuller faster, preventing overeating.
- **Put Down Your Utensils**: Take breaks between bites to allow your body time to register fullness cues. Resist the urge to clean your plate or continue eating if you're no longer hungry.
- **Identify Your Hunger and Fullness Cues**: Learn to differentiate between true hunger (physical signs like stomach growling) and emotional cues that may be disguised as hunger. Eat when you're truly hungry and

stop when you're comfortably full, not
stuffed.

- **Non-Judgmental Awareness**: Observe your thoughts and feelings surrounding food without judgment. If you find yourself criticizing yourself for certain food choices, acknowledge the thought and move on.

Mindful Eating in Everyday Life:

- **Mindful Grocery Shopping**: Plan your meals and snacks before heading to the grocery store. Create a shopping list and stick to it, avoiding impulse purchases. Read food labels and choose whole, unprocessed foods whenever possible.

- **Mindful Meal Planning**: Take some time each week to plan your meals and snacks for the upcoming days. This will help you make healthy choices and avoid unhealthy temptations when you're short on time.

- **Mindful Snacking**: Don't mindlessly reach for snacks throughout the day. Pause, ask yourself if you're truly hungry, and choose healthy, portion-controlled snacks when necessary.

- **Mindful Cooking**: Engage in the cooking process! Pay attention to the ingredients you're using and appreciate the creation of a healthy meal.

- **Mindful Eating Out**: Dining out doesn't have to derail your weight loss goals. Practice mindful eating principles by choosing healthier menu options, controlling portion sizes, and savoring each bite.

Mindful Eating Challenges and Solutions:
- **Mindless Eating**: We all fall into autopilot sometimes. If you catch yourself eating mindlessly, gently redirect your attention to the present moment and refocus on your food.
- **Emotional Eating**: If you find yourself using food to cope with stress or emotions, explore healthier coping mechanisms like exercise, journaling, or talking to a friend.
- **Time Constraints**: Even with a busy schedule, you can practice mindful eating. Pack healthy snacks and lunches to avoid unhealthy fast food options. Set a timer for 10-15 minutes to ensure you're not rushing through your meals.
- **Social Eating**: Social gatherings often involve rich food and tempting desserts. Practice mindful eating principles by

choosing smaller portions, focusing on conversation over food, and savoring each bite.

- **Negative Self-Talk:** If you find yourself criticizing yourself for your food choices, challenge those negative thoughts. Practice self-compassion and focus on progress, not perfection.

Mindful Eating Exercises:

- **The Raisin Meditation:** This simple exercise helps you focus on the sensory experience of eating. Take a single raisin and examine its appearance, smell, and texture. Slowly place it in your mouth and chew thoroughly, noticing the different flavors and sensations as you break it down. Swallow mindfully and savor the aftertaste before taking another raisin.
- **The Body Scan Meditation:** Before a meal, sit comfortably and take a few deep breaths. Focus on your body and scan from head to toe, noticing any areas of tension or discomfort. Pay attention to any hunger cues without judgment. Proceed with your meal while keeping your body awareness present.

- **The Gratitude Meal Meditation:** Before starting your meal, take a moment to express gratitude for the food in front of you. Consider the people who helped bring the food to your table, from farmers and producers to cooks and servers. Appreciate the nourishment you're about to receive and enjoy your meal with a sense of thankfulness.

Additional Tips for Cultivating Mindful Eating:

- **Keep a Mindful Eating Journal:** Track your eating habits, including what you eat, when you eat, how you feel before, during, and after eating. This can help you identify patterns and triggers for unhealthy eating habits.
- **Take Mindful Eating Classes:** Many online resources and local community centers offer mindfulness and mindful eating classes. These programs can provide additional guidance and support in developing your mindful eating practice.
- **Practice Mindfulness Throughout the Day:** Mindfulness is a skill that can be applied beyond eating. Practice mindfulness throughout the day by focusing on your breath, body sensations, and thoughts in the

present moment. This will enhance your overall awareness and improve your mindful eating practice.

Remember: Mindful eating is a journey, not a destination. There will be times when you fall back into old habits. The key is to be gentle with yourself, acknowledge the slip-up, and recommit to mindful eating practices. As you become more mindful of your relationship with food, you'll gain a sense of control and make healthier choices that support your weight loss goals and overall well-being. By incorporating these mindful eating practices into your 90-day journey, you'll be well on your way to achieving lasting weight loss success and a healthier, happier you.

Positive Affirmations: Boost Motivation and Self-Belief for Weight Loss Success (Without the Gym!)

Shedding unwanted pounds can feel like an uphill battle, especially without the traditional gym routine. But the truth is, a significant portion of weight loss success stems from your mindset. This subchapter dives into the power of positive affirmations and how they can fuel your motivation, bolster self-belief, and propel you towards achieving your 90-day weight loss goals – all from the comfort of your own home.

What are Positive Affirmations?

Positive affirmations are powerful statements that counter negative self-talk and replace it with empowering beliefs. By repeating these affirmations consistently, you can gradually shift your inner dialogue and cultivate a more positive outlook on your weight loss journey.

Why are Positive Affirmations Important for Weight Loss?

Here's how positive affirmations can significantly impact your success:

- **Boost Motivation:** When faced with challenges, negative self-talk can easily derail your efforts. But affirmations like "I am strong and capable" or "I am motivated to make healthy choices" can reignite your enthusiasm and propel you forward.
- **Enhance Self-Belief:** Doubt often lurks around the corner, whispering "you can't do this." Regularly repeating affirmations like "I am worthy of achieving my goals" or "I believe in my ability to lose weight" builds a

foundation of self-belief that empowers you to overcome limitations.

- **Promote Positive Habits:** Affirmations like "I choose healthy meals to nourish my body" or "I am committed to daily movement" can nudge you towards making positive lifestyle changes that contribute to weight loss.
- **Increase Resilience:** Setbacks are inevitable. However, affirmations like "I learn from my mistakes and keep going" or "I bounce back stronger than before" can equip you with the mental fortitude to navigate setbacks and stay committed to your journey.

How to Use Positive Affirmations Effectively
For positive affirmations to be truly effective, they need to resonate with you. Here's how to personalize and harness their power:

- **Identify Your Limiting Beliefs:** What negative self-talk holds you back? Are you afraid of failure? Do you doubt your ability to stick with a plan? Once you identify these beliefs, craft affirmations that directly contradict them.
- **Tailor Your Affirmations:** Generic affirmations like "I am a good person" can be

a good starting point. However, for a deeper impact, personalize them to your specific goals.

- **Present Tense is Powerful**: Frame your affirmations in the present tense, as if your goal is already being achieved. For example, instead of "I will be healthy," say "I am choosing healthy habits." This reinforces your commitment and belief in your ability to succeed.

- **Focus on Action & Positive Emotions**: Include action verbs and positive emotions in your affirmations. Instead of "I want to lose weight," say "I am actively taking steps towards a healthier, fitter me." This reinforces the positive feelings associated with your goals.

- **Repeat, Repeat, Repeat**: Repetition is key! Make reciting your affirmations a daily ritual. Repeat them when you wake up, before a workout, or during moments of self-doubt. Write them down, say them aloud in front of the mirror, or post them around your home – visual reminders work wonders!

Sample Positive Affirmations for Weight Loss (Without the Gym):

General Motivation:

- I am strong and capable of achieving my weight loss goals.
- I am motivated to make healthy choices for my body.
- Today is a new day, and I am choosing health and well-being.
- Every challenge presents an opportunity for growth.
- I am worthy of a healthy and vibrant life.

Focus on Action and Progress:

- I am committed to taking small, consistent steps towards my weight loss goals.
- I celebrate all my achievements, big and small.
- I choose delicious and nutritious foods that nourish my body.
- I am getting stronger and more capable with every workout.
- Every day, I am getting closer to my ideal weight.

Overcoming Setbacks and Self-Doubt:

- I learn from my mistakes and keep moving forward.

- I am strong enough to overcome challenges and setbacks.
- I believe in my ability to bounce back stronger than before.
- It takes time and effort, but I am patient with myself on this journey.
- I am worthy of self-compassion and understanding.

Embracing Healthy Habits:
- I choose to move my body in ways that make me feel good.
- I am grateful for my body and its incredible potential.
- I love nourishing myself with whole, healthy foods.
- I am creating positive habits that will last a lifetime.
- I am building a sustainable lifestyle for long-term health.

Overcoming Plateaus: Strategies to Breakthrough Weight Loss Stalls

Hitting a plateau is a common experience in any weight loss journey. It can be frustrating to see the numbers on the scale stop budging, even when you're sticking to your plan. But fear not! Plateaus are temporary, and there are strategies you can employ to break through them and keep your weight loss moving in the right direction.

Understanding Plateaus:
- **Metabolic Adaptation**: As you lose weight, your body becomes more efficient at using energy. This means you may need to adjust your calorie intake or exercise routine to keep burning calories at a higher rate.
- **Inconsistent Tracking**: Be honest with yourself – are you accurately tracking your food and activity every day? Even small slip-ups can add up and stall your progress.
- **Muscle Loss**: While losing weight, you may also lose some muscle mass. Muscle burns more calories at rest than fat, so this can slow down your metabolism.

Strategies to Break Through Your Plateau: Diet:
- **Calorie Reassessment**: Recalculate your daily calorie needs based on your current weight and activity level. A slight reduction (around 100-200 calories) might be necessary.

- **Macro Makeover**: Consider adjusting your macronutrient intake (carbs, protein, fat). Experiment with slightly lower carbs or higher protein to see if it impacts your progress.
- **Spice Up Your Meals**: Incorporate spices like cayenne pepper or chili flakes, which can boost metabolism slightly and add flavor without extra calories.
- **Hydration Hero**: Ensure you're drinking enough water throughout the day. Dehydration can sometimes mimic hunger pangs.

Exercise:
- **Intensity Increase**: If you've been sticking to a moderate-intensity routine, try adding short bursts of high-intensity interval training (HIIT) to your workouts. HIIT can boost your metabolism and calorie burn for hours after exercise.
- **Strength Training Focus**: Building muscle mass increases your resting metabolic rate, helping you burn more calories even at rest. Include bodyweight exercises, resistance bands, or free weights in your routine.

- **Shake Up Your Routine**: Prevent boredom and keep your body challenged by trying new workout styles like dance fitness, swimming, or yoga.

Lifestyle:

- **Prioritize Sleep**: Aim for 7-8 hours of quality sleep each night. Sleep deprivation can disrupt hormones that regulate hunger and metabolism.
- **Stress Less**: Chronic stress can lead to cortisol spikes, a hormone that promotes fat storage. Manage stress through relaxation techniques like deep breathing, meditation, or spending time in nature.
- **Track and Reflect**: Keep a food journal and track your progress (measurements, photos, how your clothes fit). Seeing non-scale victories can be motivating.

Bonus Tips:

- **Consider Intermittent Fasting**: This eating pattern cycles between periods of eating and fasting. Research suggests it can be effective for weight loss and metabolic health, but consult your doctor before starting.
- **Increase Accountability**: Find a weight loss buddy or join a support group. Sharing your

goals and struggles can make a big difference.

- **Celebrate Non-Scale Victories**: Focus on how you feel – more energy, better sleep, improved mood. These are all signs you're on the right track.

Remember: Plateaus are temporary setbacks, not roadblocks. By implementing these strategies and staying consistent, you can overcome them and continue your weight loss journey towards your 90-day goal!

Chapter 5:

Sleep and Recovery: The Unsung Heroes of Weight Loss

Many people underestimate the importance of sleep and recovery when it comes to weight loss. But getting enough quality shut-eye and prioritizing rest are crucial components of a successful weight loss journey, even if you're not hitting the gym. Here's why sleep matters and how to optimize your sleep routine for weight loss success.

The Science of Sleep and Weight Loss:
- **Hormonal Harmony**: Sleep regulates hormones like leptin (promotes satiety) and ghrelin (stimulates hunger). When sleep-deprived, leptin levels drop, and ghrelin rises, making you crave unhealthy foods.
- **Metabolic Boost**: During deep sleep, your body releases growth hormone, which helps build muscle and repair tissues. Muscle mass burns more calories at rest, aiding weight loss.
- **Reduced Cravings**: Sleep deprivation can impair impulse control, making you more likely to indulge in unhealthy cravings.
- **Improved Energy Levels**: Adequate sleep provides the energy you need for daily activities and exercise, which contributes to calorie burning.

Optimizing Your Sleep for Weight Loss:
Creating a Sleep Sanctuary:
- **Environment**: Ensure your bedroom is dark, cool, and quiet. Invest in blackout curtains, a comfortable mattress, and earplugs if necessary.

- **Routine**: Establish a regular sleep schedule, going to bed and waking up at consistent times, even on weekends. This regulates your body's natural sleep-wake cycle.
- **Pre-Sleep Rituals**: Develop a relaxing bedtime routine that signals to your body it's time to wind down. This could include taking a warm bath, reading a book, or practicing light stretches.

Electronics Detox:

- **Blue Light Blocker**: The blue light emitted from electronic devices like phones and laptops can disrupt sleep patterns. Avoid using them for at least an hour before bed or use blue light-blocking glasses.
- **Power Down Early**: Turn off electronic devices in your bedroom. The constant notifications and temptation to check social media can disrupt sleep.

Habit Hacks for Better Sleep:

- **Regular Exercise**: Physical activity promotes better sleep quality, but avoid strenuous workouts too close to bedtime.
- **Light Dinner**: Avoid heavy meals close to bedtime, as they can cause indigestion and

disrupt sleep. Opt for a light, healthy dinner at least 2-3 hours before sleep.

- **Relaxation Techniques**: Practice relaxation techniques like deep breathing, meditation, or progressive muscle relaxation before bed to calm your mind and body.
- **Limited Caffeine and Alcohol**: While a morning coffee might be your ritual, limit caffeine intake later in the day as it can interfere with sleep. Avoid alcohol close to bedtime, as it disrupts sleep patterns.

Addressing Sleep Issues:

- **Identify the Cause**: Are you struggling to fall asleep, stay asleep, or experience restless sleep? Identifying the root cause can help you address it effectively.
- **Seek Professional Help**: If you're consistently experiencing sleep problems, consult a doctor to rule out any underlying medical conditions and get personalized advice.

Remember: Prioritizing sleep is an investment in your overall health and weight loss goals. By making these adjustments and creating a sleep-supportive environment, you'll be well on your way to achieving restful nights and successful weight loss, all without a gym membership!

Quality Sleep: The Powerhouse Behind Weight Loss

We all know the importance of a good night's sleep. But when it comes to weight loss, sleep often takes a backseat to diet and exercise. However, research reveals that quality sleep is a **powerhouse** behind successful weight loss, even when you're not hitting the gym. Here's a deep dive into why sleep matters so much for shedding pounds.

The Hormonal Symphony:

Our bodies are complex ecosystems, and sleep plays a vital role in regulating hormones that directly impact weight management. During sleep, a delicate hormonal dance occurs:

- **Leptin (the satiety hormone):** Levels of leptin, which signals feeling full, rise during sleep. When sleep-deprived, leptin levels **plummet**, leaving you feeling hungrier and more likely to overeat.

- **Ghrelin (the hunger hormone):** Sleep deprivation triggers a surge in ghrelin, the hormone that stimulates hunger. This makes you crave unhealthy, calorie-dense foods, hindering your weight loss efforts.
- **Cortisol (the stress hormone):** Chronic sleep deprivation elevates cortisol levels. Cortisol promotes fat storage, especially around the abdomen, contributing to weight gain.

Metabolic Marvels:

Sleep isn't just about feeling refreshed; it's a time for your body to **repair and rebuild**. Here's how sleep fuels your metabolism for weight loss:

- **Growth Hormone:** Deep sleep triggers the release of growth hormone, which plays a crucial role in building and repairing muscle tissue. Muscle burns more calories at rest than fat, so having more muscle mass naturally boosts your metabolism and calorie burning potential.
- **Insulin Sensitivity:** Adequate sleep improves your body's sensitivity to insulin, a hormone responsible for regulating blood sugar levels. Improved insulin sensitivity allows your body to use glucose (sugar) for energy more

efficiently, preventing it from being stored as fat.

Beyond Hormones and Metabolism:

Sleep's impact on weight loss extends beyond hormones and metabolism. Here's how:

- **Curbs Cravings:** Sleep deprivation impairs your impulse control, making you more susceptible to giving in to unhealthy cravings and sabotaging your weight loss goals.
- **Boosts Energy Levels:** A good night's sleep provides sustained energy throughout the day. You'll be more motivated to make healthy choices and engage in physical activity, which contributes to calorie burning.
- **Improves Decision-Making:** Sleep deprivation affects your cognitive function, making it harder to make healthy food choices and stick to your weight loss plan.

The Takeaway:

Quality sleep is an essential, yet often overlooked, pillar of a successful weight loss journey. By understanding how sleep regulates hormones, boosts your metabolism, and empowers healthy choices, you can harness its power to achieve your 90-day weight loss goal without relying on a gym membership. Prioritizing sleep is an investment in your overall health and a key to unlocking lasting weight loss success.

Rest Days: The Importance of Allowing Your Body to Rebuild and Recharge

While pushing yourself and staying active are important for weight loss, neglecting rest days can be counterproductive. Just like a car needs regular maintenance to run smoothly, your body requires dedicated recovery time to function optimally and optimize your weight loss journey. Here's why rest days are crucial, even when you're not following a gym-based routine.

The Science Behind Rest Days:

Muscle Repair and Growth: Exercise, especially intense workouts, creates microscopic tears in your muscle fibers. Rest days allow your body to focus on repairing these tears, leading to stronger, more resilient muscles. This muscle-building process is essential for boosting your metabolism, as muscle burns more calories at rest compared to fat.

Replenishing Energy Stores: During exercise, your body utilizes glycogen, its primary source of readily available energy, stored in your muscles and liver. Rest days provide an opportunity for your body to replenish these glycogen stores, ensuring you have the energy you need to tackle your next workout and daily activities.

Hormonal Harmony: Strenuous exercise can lead to increased levels of cortisol, the stress hormone. Chronically elevated cortisol levels can hinder weight loss by promoting fat storage and disrupting your sleep-wake cycle. Rest days allow cortisol levels to return to normal, promoting a hormonal environment conducive to weight loss.

Preventing Injuries: Pushing yourself too hard without rest days increases your risk of overuse injuries. These injuries can force you to take a longer break from exercise, stalling your weight loss progress. Rest days give your muscles and joints time to recover, preventing injuries and allowing you to stay consistent with your weight loss efforts.

Mental and Emotional Benefits: Rest days aren't just about physical recovery; they're crucial for mental and emotional well-being too. A constant state of exertion can lead to burnout and demotivation. Rest days allow you to recharge mentally, making you more likely to stick with your weight loss plan in the long run.

How Many Rest Days Do You Need?

The ideal number of rest days depends on various factors, including your overall fitness level, the intensity of your workouts, and your body's recovery rate. Here's a general guideline:

- **Beginners:** Aim for 1-2 rest days per week.
- **Intermediate:** Consider 2-3 rest days per week.
- **Advanced:** Experienced exercisers may require only 1 rest day per week, but it's still important to listen to your body and take additional rest when needed.

Making the Most of Your Rest Days:

Rest days don't have to mean being completely sedentary. Here are some ideas for active recovery that can further enhance your weight loss journey:

- **Low-Intensity Activities**: Go for a walk, do some gentle yoga or stretching, or try a light swim. These activities keep your blood flowing and promote recovery without putting undue stress on your body.
- **Focus on Self-Care**: Get a massage, take a relaxing bath, or practice mindfulness techniques. Prioritizing self-care helps manage stress and promotes better sleep, both of which are beneficial for weight loss.
- **Healthy Eating**: Don't let your rest days turn into cheat days. Stick to your healthy eating plan to fuel your body's recovery process and avoid weight gain.

Remember: Rest days are not a sign of weakness; they're a crucial part of a successful weight loss journey. By incorporating rest days into your routine, you'll allow your body to recover, rebuild, and recharge, leading to optimal weight loss results and a healthier, more energized you.

Stress Management: Techniques to Reduce Stress-Related Weight Gain

Stress is a fact of life, but it can wreak havoc on your weight loss efforts. When stressed, your body releases cortisol, a hormone that promotes fat storage, particularly around the belly. Additionally, stress can lead to unhealthy coping mechanisms like emotional eating and neglecting exercise, hindering weight loss progress.

The good news is that there are effective stress management techniques you can integrate into your daily routine, even without a gym membership, to combat stress-related weight gain and support your 90-day weight loss goal.

Understanding the Stress-Weight Gain Connection:

- **Cortisol and Cravings:** Cortisol not only promotes fat storage but also triggers cravings for sugary and high-fat foods, often seen as comfort foods during stressful times. These calorie-dense options can sabotage your weight loss efforts.
- **Disrupted Sleep:** Chronic stress disrupts sleep patterns, making it harder to fall asleep and stay asleep. Sleep deprivation, as

you learned earlier, can further disrupt hormones and increase cravings, leading to weight gain.

- **Reduced Motivation:** Stress can zap your motivation to exercise and prioritize healthy eating habits. You may find yourself skipping workouts or resorting to quick, unhealthy meals due to a lack of energy and mental clarity.

Stress Management Techniques for Weight Loss Success:

Mindfulness and Relaxation:

- **Meditation:** Regular meditation practice can help calm your mind, reduce stress hormones, and improve sleep quality. There are many guided meditation apps and resources available to help you get started.
- **Deep Breathing Exercises:** Taking slow, deep breaths activates your body's relaxation response, counteracting the stress response. Practice deep breathing throughout the day, especially during stressful situations.
- **Progressive Muscle Relaxation:** This technique involves tensing and relaxing

different muscle groups one at a time, promoting relaxation and stress relief.

Physical Activity for Stress Reduction:

- **Walking:** Even a brisk walk outdoors can work wonders for reducing stress and improving mood. Walking in nature has additional benefits as it exposes you to sunlight and fresh air.
- **Yoga:** Yoga combines physical postures, breathing exercises, and meditation, offering a holistic approach to stress management. Many styles of yoga are suitable for beginners, and there are numerous online yoga classes available.
- **Tai Chi:** This gentle exercise form incorporates slow, deliberate movements that promote relaxation, improve balance, and reduce stress.

Lifestyle Modifications for Stress Management:

- **Prioritize Sleep:** As discussed earlier, sleep is crucial for stress management and weight loss. Aim for 7-8 hours of quality sleep each night.
- **Healthy Eating:** Fuel your body with nutritious foods that provide sustained

energy. Focus on fruits, vegetables, whole grains, and lean protein sources to manage stress effectively.

- **Limit Caffeine and Alcohol:** While a morning coffee might be your ritual, excessive caffeine intake can exacerbate anxiety and stress. Similarly, alcohol might provide a temporary sense of relaxation but disrupts sleep and contributes to weight gain in the long run.
- **Connect with Loved Ones:** Social support plays a vital role in stress management. Spend time with friends and family who uplift and encourage you, and don't be afraid to ask for help when needed.
- **Identify Your Stressors:** Being aware of your triggers allows you to develop strategies for coping with stressful situations in a healthy way.

Bonus Tip: Consider journaling or talking to a therapist to explore your stress triggers and develop coping mechanisms specific to your needs.

Remember, managing stress is an ongoing process. Experiment with different techniques and find what works best for you. By incorporating these stress management strategies into your routine, you'll be well on your way to reducing stress-related weight gain and achieving your 90-day weight loss goal. You'll not only see results on the scale but also feel calmer, more energized, and empowered to handle life's challenges in a healthy way.

Chapter 6

Tracking Progress and Adjustments - Mastering Your 90-Day Weight Loss Journey

Congratulations! You've embarked on your 90-day weight loss journey, armed with valuable knowledge about healthy eating, exercise strategies without a gym, and the importance of sleep and stress management. But reaching your goal requires consistency, monitoring progress, and making adjustments along the way. This chapter will equip you with powerful tools for tracking your progress and making data-driven adjustments to maximize success.

Why Track Your Progress?

Tracking your progress is like having a roadmap for your weight loss journey. It provides valuable insights into your efforts, keeps you motivated, and helps identify areas where adjustments might be necessary. Here's how tracking can benefit you:

- **Accountability:** Recording your daily food intake, exercise routines, and weight measurements creates a sense of accountability. Knowing you'll be tracking your progress motivates you to stick to your plan and make healthy choices.
- **Motivation Booster:** Seeing the numbers on the scale decrease can be incredibly

motivating. But weight loss isn't always linear. Tracking other metrics like body measurements, increased energy levels, and improved sleep can be even more motivating when the scale seems stagnant.

- **Identification of Trends**: Tracking allows you to analyze trends over time. You might notice specific foods or activities that lead to bloating or energy dips. This knowledge allows for adjustments and personalization of your plan.
- **Celebrating Milestones**: Tracking progress helps you appreciate the smaller victories, not just the final destination. Celebrate reaching milestones, like losing your first few pounds or completing a week of consistent exercise.

What to Track:
- **Food Intake**: This doesn't require calorie counting at the beginning. Start by simply tracking what you eat and drink throughout the day. There are several methods for this:
  - **Food Journal**: Keep a notebook or use a dedicated app to record everything you consume, including portion sizes.

- Photo Journal: Capture images of your meals to visualize portion sizes and identify areas for improvement.
- **Weight**: Weigh yourself regularly, ideally first thing in the morning after using the restroom and before eating or drinking anything. Track your weight weekly or bi-weekly to avoid obsessing over daily fluctuations.
- **Body Measurements**: Weight isn't the only indicator of progress. Measuring key body parts like your chest, waist, hips, and thighs allows you to see how your body composition is changing, even if the scale doesn't always reflect it immediately.
- **Activity Level**: Track your daily activity levels, including any workouts you perform (duration, intensity), steps taken throughout the day, or participation in active hobbies.
- **Sleep**: Monitor your sleep patterns by recording the time you fall asleep, wake up, and the quality of your sleep (restful, restless). This allows you to identify potential sleep issues that might be hindering your weight loss efforts.
- **Mood and Energy Levels**: Track your overall mood and energy levels throughout the day.

This can help you identify patterns and adjust your diet or activity routines to optimize energy levels and combat stress.

Tracking Tools and Resources:
- **Food Tracking Apps:** Numerous free and paid apps like MyFitnessPal, Lose It!, and MyPlate make food logging easy and convenient.
- **Weight Tracking Apps:** Simple apps like Libra or Weight Tracker can help you monitor your weight and analyze trends over time.
- **Body Measurement Apps:** Some apps like Bodyscale or Caliper can help you track and visualize body composition changes.
- **Fitness Trackers:** Wearable fitness trackers can monitor your daily activity levels, sleep patterns, and even heart rate, providing valuable insights into your overall health and fitness.
- **Printable Trackers:** If you prefer a non-digital approach, you can find printable food and activity trackers online.

Making Data-Driven Adjustments:

Tracking provides valuable data to guide your adjustments. Here's how to use that data effectively:

- **Reviewing Progress**: Regularly review your tracked data. Are you sticking to your calorie intake goals? Is your activity level sufficient? How are your sleep patterns?
- **Identifying Trends**: Look for patterns in your data. Are there specific foods causing bloating? Do certain workout routines leave you feeling depleted?
- **Adjusting Your Plan**: Based on your data and trends, consider making adjustments to your plan. This might involve tweaking your calorie intake, modifying your exercise routines, incorporating more stress management techniques, or prioritizing sleep hygiene.
- **Seeking Support**: Don't be afraid to seek support from a registered dietitian, certified personal trainer, or health coach if you need help interpreting your data or making impactful adjustments.

Beyond the Numbers:

While tracking has tremendous value, remember it's about more than just numbers on a scale or app. Here are some important considerations:

- **Focus on How You Feel**: Weight loss isn't just about aesthetics; it's about feeling your best. Track your energy levels, mood, sleep quality, and overall well-being. Notice if you have increased stamina, improved sleep, or a more positive outlook. These qualitative measures are equally important indicators of progress.
- **Celebrate Non-Scale Victories**: Don't get discouraged if the scale doesn't always move as quickly as you'd like. Celebrate non-scale victories like fitting into old clothes comfortably, having more energy for daily activities, or experiencing fewer aches and pains.
- **Listen to Your Body**: Tracking can help you identify food sensitivities or activities that trigger discomfort. Listen to your body's cues and adjust your plan accordingly. Don't push yourself to the point of exhaustion or injury.

Maintaining Consistency:

Tracking and adjustments are crucial, but consistency is the key to achieving and maintaining your weight loss goals. Here are some tips for staying consistent throughout your 90-day journey:

- **Set SMART Goals:** Make your goals Specific, Measurable, Achievable, Relevant, and Time-bound. Instead of a vague goal of "losing weight," set a goal like "losing 1 pound per week for the next 12 weeks."
- **Plan Your Meals:** Planning healthy meals and snacks in advance helps you avoid unhealthy choices when you're feeling hungry or rushed.
- **Find an Exercise Routine You Enjoy:** If you hate running, don't force yourself to do it. Choose activities you find enjoyable, whether it's dancing, swimming, brisk walking, or bodyweight exercises at home.
- **Schedule Your Workouts:** Treat your workouts like important appointments and schedule them in your calendar. This increases the likelihood of sticking to your routine.
- **Find an Accountability Partner:** Partner with a friend or family member who shares similar weight loss goals. You can motivate and support each other throughout the journey.

Remember: Weight loss is a journey, not a destination. There will be setbacks and plateaus along the way. Use tracking data to make adjustments, celebrate your victories, and focus on how you feel. By staying consistent, flexible, and prioritizing your overall well-being, you'll be well on your way to achieving your 90-day weight loss goal and developing healthy habits for a lifetime. This book equips you with the knowledge and tools to transform your life, not just for the next 90 days, but for a healthier, happier you!

Food Journaling - Keeping Track of Your Meals and Progress

Food journaling is a powerful tool for anyone embarking on a weight loss journey, especially when following a non-gym-based approach. It allows you to gain valuable insights into your eating habits, identify areas for improvement, and track your progress towards your 90-day weight loss goal. Here's a comprehensive guide to utilizing food journaling effectively:

Benefits of Food Journaling:
- **Increased Awareness:** The simple act of writing down everything you eat and drink

throughout the day fosters awareness. You'll be more mindful of your portion sizes, snacking habits, and the types of foods you're consuming. This awareness is crucial for making informed choices and developing healthy eating patterns.

- **Identifying Triggers**: Tracking your food intake can help you identify potential triggers for unhealthy eating habits. Are you more likely to reach for sugary snacks when stressed? Does boredom lead to mindless munching? Recognizing these triggers empowers you to develop coping mechanisms and make healthier substitutions.

- **Spotting Nutritional Imbalances**: By recording food details, you can identify potential nutritional gaps in your diet. Are you lacking in fruits or vegetables? Is your protein intake insufficient? This knowledge allows you to adjust your meals to ensure you're getting the essential nutrients your body needs.

- **Tracking Progress**: Food journaling helps you track your progress beyond just the scale. You might notice specific foods causing bloating or low energy levels. Additionally, recording portion sizes can help you visualize your calorie intake and make adjustments as needed.

How to Get Started with Food Journaling:

There's no one-size-fits-all approach to food journaling. Choose a method that works best for you:

- **Pen and Paper**: This classic method provides flexibility and allows you to capture additional notes about your mood, hunger levels, or any physical reactions to certain foods.
- **Food Tracking Apps**: Numerous free and paid apps like MyFitnessPal, Lose It!, and MyPlate simplify food logging. They offer extensive food databases, calorie tracking tools, and progress charts.
- **Photo Journaling**: Taking pictures of your meals can be a helpful visual aid for portion control and identifying patterns in your food choices.

What to Include in Your Food Journal:
- **Time**: Record the time of each meal and snack. This helps you identify potential

patterns in your eating habits and areas for improvement.

- **Food and Beverage Details:** Be specific about what you consume, including the type of food, portion size, and brand (if applicable). This allows for a more accurate analysis of your calorie intake and nutrient content.
- **Preparation Method:** Note how your food is prepared (baked, fried, grilled) as cooking methods can significantly impact calorie content and healthfulness.
- **Hunger Level:** Before each meal or snack, record your hunger level on a scale (e.g., 1-10). This helps you distinguish between true hunger and emotional or mindless eating.
- **Mood and Energy Levels:** Jot down your mood and energy levels throughout the day. This can reveal a connection between certain foods and your overall well-being.
- **Additional Notes:** Feel free to include any additional notes relevant to your weight loss journey. Did you experience any food sensitivities? Did a particular meal leave you feeling sluggish? These details can provide valuable insights.

Tips for Effective Food Journaling:

- **Be Honest and Consistent:** The key to success is honesty and consistency. Track everything you consume, even if you feel embarrassed or discouraged. The more accurate your data, the more valuable it becomes.
- **Don't Obsess Over Perfection:** Food journaling isn't about micromanaging every calorie. Aim for consistency and focus on developing healthy eating habits.
- **Review Regularly:** Schedule regular periods to review your food journal entries. Look for patterns, identify areas for improvement, and adjust your meal plan accordingly.
- **Celebrate Non-Scale Victories:** Food journaling helps you recognize victories beyond the scale. Did you choose a healthier option over a processed snack? Did you increase your fruit and vegetable intake? Celebrate these positive changes!
- **Seek Help if Needed:** A registered dietitian can help you analyze your food journal entries and create a meal plan tailored to your specific needs and goals.

By incorporating food journaling into your 90-day weight loss journey, you'll gain powerful insights into your eating habits, make informed choices, and achieve your weight loss goals in a healthy and sustainable way. Remember, food journaling is a tool for self-awareness and positive change. Embrace the process, and use the information you gather to cultivate a healthier relationship with food and achieve lasting weight loss success.

Weekly Assessments - Evaluating Your Weight Loss Journey and Making Adjustments

Regular evaluation is crucial for any successful endeavor, and your 90-day weight loss journey is no exception. Weekly assessments allow you to track your progress, identify areas for improvement, and make adjustments to your plan as needed. This proactive approach ensures you stay on track and achieve your weight loss goals.

Benefits of Weekly Assessments:
- **Progress Tracking:** Weekly assessments go beyond simply checking the scale. You'll evaluate various metrics to gain a more comprehensive understanding of your progress. This holistic approach allows you to celebrate victories and identify areas where your plan needs tweaking.

- **Identifying Trends**: Regular assessments help you identify trends over time. Are you consistently losing weight? Is your sleep improving? Are there specific activities that leave you depleted? Analyzing these trends allows for targeted adjustments and ensures your plan remains effective.
- **Staying Motivated**: Seeing progress, however small, can be incredibly motivating. Weekly assessments provide a chance to acknowledge your victories and recommit to your goals. This can be particularly beneficial when facing plateaus or setbacks.
- **Adaptability**: Your body's needs and responses may change throughout your journey. Weekly assessments allow you to adapt your plan accordingly. This flexibility ensures you can maintain progress and avoid feeling discouraged by a rigid approach.

What to Assess Each Week:
- **Weight**: Weigh yourself once a week, ideally first thing in the morning after using the restroom and before eating or drinking anything. Track your weight to monitor progress, but remember, weight loss isn't

always linear. Don't get discouraged by minor fluctuations.

- **Body Measurements:** Track key body parts like your chest, waist, hips, and thighs. Measuring allows you to see how your body composition is changing, even if the scale doesn't reflect it immediately.
- **Activity Level:** Assess your activity level for the past week. Did you stick to your exercise routine? Did you incorporate additional movement throughout the day? Analyze your activity levels and adjust your plan as needed.
- **Food Intake:** Review your food journal entries from the week. Did you stick to your planned meals and snacks? Did you encounter any challenges or areas for improvement? Use this review to refine your meal plan for the upcoming week.
- **Sleep Quality:** Evaluate your sleep patterns for the past week. Did you get enough restful sleep? Are there any factors affecting your sleep quality? Address any sleep issues to ensure you're getting the restorative sleep needed for optimal weight loss and overall health.

- **Energy Levels and Mood**: Track your overall energy levels and mood throughout the week. Are your energy levels consistent? Has your mood improved? This can reveal potential connections between food choices, activity levels, and well-being.

Making Adjustments Based on Your Assessments:

After analyzing your weekly assessments, it's time to make adjustments to your plan as needed. Here's how:

- **Maintaining What Works**: If you're seeing progress and feeling good, stick with what's working! Consistency is key to achieving your weight loss goals.
- **Tweaking Your Food Plan**: Based on your food journal entries, adjust your calorie intake or meal composition if needed. Perhaps you need to increase your protein intake or incorporate more fruits and vegetables.
- **Modifying Your Exercise Routine**: If you're not seeing results or find your workouts too easy, increase the intensity or duration of your workouts. If you're feeling

overwhelmed, consider adding more rest days or modifying the intensity.

- **Prioritizing Sleep:** If your sleep quality is lacking, identify the root cause and implement strategies to improve sleep hygiene. This could involve establishing a regular sleep schedule, creating a relaxing bedtime routine, or addressing any underlying sleep disorders.
- **Stress Management Techniques:** If stress is hindering your progress, incorporate stress management techniques like meditation, deep breathing exercises, or yoga into your routine.

Additional Tips for Effective Weekly Assessments:

- **Schedule Assessments:** Set aside a specific time each week to conduct your assessments. This helps you stay consistent and ensures you're taking a holistic approach to evaluate your journey.
- **Track Your Notes:** Keep a dedicated notebook or app to track your assessments and adjustments over time. This allows you to see the bigger picture and identify long-term trends.

- **Celebrate Non-Scale Victories:** Beyond weight loss, celebrate non-scale victories like increased energy levels, better sleep quality, or improved mood. These positive changes are indicators of progress and contribute to overall well-being.
- **Seek Support:** Don't be afraid to seek support from a registered dietitian, certified personal trainer, or health coach. They can help you analyze your assessments, make adjustments, and stay motivated throughout your journey.

Remember: Weekly Assessments Are an Opportunity for Growth

Weekly assessments are an opportunity for growth and refinement, not a judgment of your progress. Embrace these assessments as a chance to learn from your experiences, celebrate your victories, and fine-tune your plan for success.

Here are some additional points to consider:

- **Be Patient and Kind to Yourself:** Weight loss takes time and dedication. Don't get discouraged by setbacks or plateaus.

Celebrate progress, big or small, and trust the process.

- **Focus on Sustainability:** Aim for sustainable lifestyle changes, not quick fixes. Weekly assessments help you identify habits you can maintain for long-term success.
- **Enjoy the Journey:** Focus on the positive changes you're making and the healthier habits you're cultivating. Enjoy the process of becoming a stronger, healthier you.

By incorporating weekly assessments into your 90-day weight loss journey, you'll gain valuable insights, make data-driven adjustments, and stay motivated to achieve your goals. Remember, you're not alone in this journey. Utilize the tools and resources provided in this book, seek support when needed, and believe in your ability to create lasting change. With dedication and a positive mindset, you'll reach your weight loss goals and experience a healthier, happier you!

Adaptability - The Key to Sustainable Weight Loss Success

The human body is an incredibly adaptable machine. What worked for you initially in your 90-

day weight loss journey might not continue to yield results indefinitely. This is where adaptability becomes crucial. By embracing a flexible approach and adjusting your plan based on your results, you ensure long-term success and avoid plateaus. Here's how to harness the power of adaptability for sustainable weight loss:

Understanding the Need for Adaptability:
- **Metabolic Adaptations:** As you lose weight, your body's metabolism naturally slows down to conserve energy. This can make it harder to lose weight further if you stick to the same exact plan you started with.
- **Changing Needs:** Your needs and preferences might evolve throughout your journey. Maybe you've encountered new dietary restrictions, or your exercise preferences have changed. A flexible plan allows for adjustments to accommodate these changes.
- **Plateaus:** Everyone experiences plateaus, periods where weight loss stalls despite following your plan. Adapting your approach can help break through these plateaus and keep the progress moving forward.

Strategies for Adapting Your Weight Loss Plan:

- **Monitor Your Progress**: This is where the importance of weekly assessments (discussed in Subchapter 2) comes into play. Regularly tracking your weight, body measurements, activity levels, and overall well-being allows you to identify areas where adjustments might be necessary.
- **Listen to Your Body**: Pay attention to your body's cues. Are you feeling unusually tired after your workouts? Does a specific food cause bloating or discomfort? Adjust your plan accordingly. Prioritize rest if needed, or swap out a food that triggers negative reactions.
- **Adjust Calorie Intake**: As you lose weight and your metabolism adapts, you might need to adjust your calorie intake to maintain a calorie deficit. A registered dietitian can help you determine the appropriate adjustments based on your current weight, activity level, and goals.
- **Progressing Your Workouts**: If you've been consistently following your exercise routine and haven't seen results in a while, it might be time to increase the intensity or duration of your workouts. This keeps your body challenged and helps overcome plateaus.

- **Incorporate Variety:** Doing the same exercises day in and day out can lead to boredom and a plateau in results. Introduce variety into your workouts by trying new activities, experimenting with different workout splits, or exploring outdoor activities like hiking or swimming.

Additional Tips for Adaptable Weight Loss:

- **Embrace New Challenges:** Don't be afraid to step outside your comfort zone and try new healthy recipes, explore different exercise formats, or join a fitness class.

- **Seek Support:** Having a registered dietitian or certified personal trainer on your side can be invaluable. They can help you analyze your progress, recommend adjustments to your plan, and keep you motivated.

- **Celebrate Non-Scale Victories:** Focus on celebrating non-scale victories alongside weight loss. Did you complete a workout you were previously struggling with? Are you noticing increased stamina? These achievements are a testament to your progress.

Adaptability: A Mindset Shift

Adaptability isn't just about changing your plan; it's a mindset shift. Embrace the journey with a willingness to learn, adjust, and explore different strategies. Here are some additional points to consider:

- **Focus on Progress:** Don't get fixated on achieving perfection. Celebrate any progress, no matter how small, and focus on the continuous journey towards a healthier you.
- **Learning from Setbacks:** Setbacks are inevitable. View them as an opportunity to learn what works and what doesn't for your body. Use setbacks as a springboard to refine your approach and become more resilient.
- **Enjoy the Process:** Embrace the journey of learning about your body, developing healthier habits, and becoming a stronger you. Finding joy in the process makes weight loss sustainable and fosters a lifelong commitment to well-being.

By incorporating adaptability into your 90-day weight loss journey, you'll be well-equipped to overcome challenges, break through plateaus, and achieve lasting success. Remember, weight loss is a marathon, not a sprint. Embrace flexibility, listen to your body, and enjoy the journey to a healthier, happier you!

Chapter 7

Weight Loss Supplements: A Critical Examination

The weight loss industry is bombarded with claims about miracle supplements that promise effortless fat burning and rapid weight loss. While some supplements might offer specific benefits, it's crucial to approach them with a critical eye and understand their limitations within your 90-day weight loss journey, particularly when focusing on non-gym-based strategies.

Here's a comprehensive look at weight loss supplements, their potential benefits, drawbacks, and how to navigate this often-confusing landscape:

Understanding Weight Loss Supplements:

Weight loss supplements come in various forms like pills, powders, and liquids, each containing a specific ingredient or combination of ingredients aimed at achieving various goals:

- **Appetite Suppression**: These supplements aim to curb your appetite, helping you consume fewer calories. Examples include fiber supplements like glucomannan and garcinia cambogia.
- **Fat Burning**: Some supplements claim to boost metabolism and increase the rate at which your body burns fat. Examples include green tea extract and conjugated linoleic acid (CLA).
- **Blocking Fat Absorption**: These supplements claim to prevent your body from absorbing fat from food. An example is chitosan.

The Reality of Weight Loss Supplements:

While some supplements might offer limited benefits, it's essential to manage expectations:

- **Limited Scientific Evidence**: Many weight loss supplements lack strong scientific evidence to support their effectiveness in promoting long-term, sustainable weight loss.
- **Potential Side Effects**: Some supplements can cause side effects like digestive upset, headaches, or interactions with medications. It's crucial to consult with your doctor before using any supplement.

- **Not a Magic Bullet**: Supplements should be viewed as a potential aid, not a replacement for a healthy diet and regular exercise.

Focusing on Sustainable Strategies:

Here's why a sustainable approach focusing on healthy eating and regular activity is more effective for weight loss than relying on supplements:

- **Developing Healthy Habits**: By focusing on whole, unprocessed foods, portion control, and regular exercise, you'll cultivate sustainable habits for long-term weight management and overall well-being.
- **Addressing the Root Cause**: Supplements often address symptoms (weight gain) but not the root cause (unhealthy eating habits or lack of physical activity). Focus on building a healthy lifestyle for lasting change.
- **Building a Foundation**: A sustainable approach teaches you valuable tools for managing your weight in the long run. Supplements often offer a temporary solution.

Alternatives to Weight Loss Supplements:

Instead of relying on supplements, consider incorporating these strategies into your weight loss journey:

- **Fiber-Rich Foods**: Fiber promotes satiety and helps you feel fuller for longer, aiding in weight management. Focus on whole grains, fruits, vegetables, and legumes to increase your fiber intake.
- **Protein Power**: Protein also promotes satiety and helps you maintain muscle mass, which can boost metabolism. Include lean protein sources like chicken, fish, beans, and lentils in your diet.
- **Mindful Eating**: Practice mindful eating by paying attention to hunger cues, savoring your food, and avoiding distractions while eating. This helps you eat intuitively and avoid overeating.
- **Staying Hydrated**: Drinking plenty of water throughout the day keeps you feeling full and can help curb cravings. Aim for eight glasses of water daily.

The Bottom Line on Supplements:

Weight loss supplements might offer some limited benefits, but they are not a magic bullet for achieving sustainable weight loss. Focus on building healthy eating habits, incorporating regular exercise, and prioritizing mindful eating practices for long-term success.

If you're considering using a supplement, consult your doctor first to discuss potential interactions with medications and ensure it's safe for you. Remember, a healthy lifestyle is the key to achieving and maintaining a healthy weight.

Conclusion

Your 90-Day Journey to a Healthier You - Without the Gym!

Congratulations! You've reached the end of your 90-day weight loss journey guide. Armed with the knowledge and tools within these pages, you're well-equipped to achieve your goals, develop healthy habits, and embark on a lifelong journey towards a healthier, happier you, all without stepping foot in a gym.

This book has emphasized the importance of **sustainable strategies**. You've learned about creating a calorie deficit through healthy eating choices, incorporating effective non-gym-based exercise routines, prioritizing sleep and stress management, and fostering a positive mindset for success.

Remember: Weight loss is a journey, not a destination. There will be bumps along the road, plateaus to overcome, and moments of temptation. Embrace adaptability, celebrate non-scale victories, and listen to your body's cues.

Here are some key takeaways to carry with you:

- **Focus on Whole Foods**: Prioritize whole, unprocessed foods like fruits, vegetables, whole grains, and lean protein sources.
- **Portion Control Matters**: Be mindful of portion sizes and find ways to manage hunger through healthy snacks, staying hydrated, and practicing mindful eating.
- **Move Your Body**: Incorporate various physical activities you enjoy into your routine, whether it's brisk walking, dancing, bodyweight exercises at home, or outdoor adventures.
- **Track Your Progress**: Food journaling and regular assessments provide valuable insights

into your efforts and empower you to personalize your plan for optimal results.

- **Prioritize Sleep**: Aim for 7-8 hours of quality sleep each night for optimal health, weight management, and stress reduction.
- **Manage Stress**: Develop healthy coping mechanisms to manage stress, a major contributor to weight gain. Explore techniques like meditation, deep breathing, yoga, or journaling.
- **Seek Support**: Surround yourself with positive and supportive individuals who share your health goals. Consider a registered dietitian, personal trainer, or health coach for additional guidance.
- **Be Patient and Kind to Yourself**: Celebrate progress, big or small, and trust the process.

Most importantly, enjoy the journey! Explore new healthy recipes, discover physical activities you actually enjoy, and celebrate the positive changes you're making to your well-being.

Remember, you are not alone. This book serves as a starting point for your lifelong journey towards a healthier you. Hold onto the knowledge you've gained, embrace challenges with resilience, and

never give up on your quest for a healthier,
happier life.

Acknowledgement

I wish to thank Almighty God for the inspiration to undertake this project and contribute to the society positively.

About the Author

Leo Chambers is a creative writer and Digital Content Creator.